DERMATOLOGY

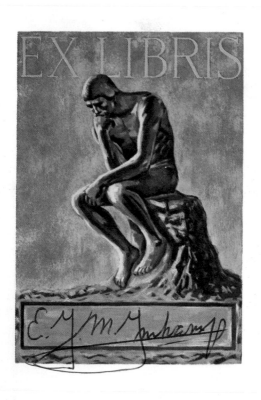

CONCISE

MEDICAL

TEXTBOOKS

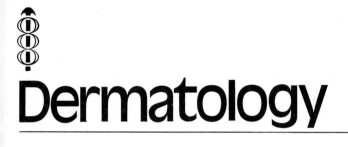

Dermatology

J. S. PEGUM
M.D., F.R.C.P.
Physician to the Skin Department,
The London Hospital;
Consultant Dermatologist to the
Queen Elizabeth Hospital for Children;
Civil Consultant in Dermatology to the
Royal Navy

HARVEY BAKER
M.D., F.R.C.P.
Physician to the Skin Department,
The London Hospital

Third Edition

BAILLIÈRE TINDALL · LONDON

A BAILLIÈRE TINDALL book published by
Cassell Ltd,
35 Red Lion Square, London WC1R 4SG
and at Sydney, Auckland, Toronto, Johannesburg
an affiliate of
Macmillan Publishing Co. Inc.
New York

© 1979 Baillière Tindall
a division of Cassell Ltd

First published 1964
Second edition 1970

Third edition 1979

ISBN 0 7020 0683 1

Printed in Great Britain by Lowe & Brydone Printers Limited,
Thetford, Norfolk

British Library Cataloguing in Publication Data

Pegum, Joseph Stephen
 Dermatology. – 3rd ed.
 – (Concise medical textbooks).
 1. Dermatology
 I. Title II. Baker, Harvey
 III. MacKenna, Robert Merttins
 Bird IV. Series
 616.5   RL71

 ISBN 0-7020-0683-1

CONTENTS

LIST OF COLOUR PLATES

(Between pages 136 and 137)

PREFACE

This textbook is addressed to medical students and to doctors of all kinds (except dermatologists). It is concerned with the basic biology of the skin and with common skin diseases. We have not hesitated to include rarities if they can illustrate a general principle or give a little bubble to what might not otherwise sparkle.

The last edition was in 1970 and we have almost entirely re-written the text, leaving here and there a telling phrase or description from the original and much admired text of Dr R. M. B. MacKenna and Dr E. L. Cohen. We have re-written because medicine alters rapidly (some would say advances) and inevitably we have surrendered some (perhaps not quite enough) of the esoteric jargon of dermatology. We have taken cognizance of advances in biology, in immunology, in diagnosis, and in therapy.

We have heeded the criticisms of the last edition. The chapters have been re-arranged and their number increased. We have altered the previous synoptic style in order to make the text easier to read. There are colour plates for the first time, and black and white pictures within the text.

We should like to thank our publishers for their co-operation and patience, Mr R. F. Ruddick and his staff of the Photographic Department of The London Hospital for most of the illustrations, and Dr J. Adamson for allowing us to print Plate V. . . .

January 1979

J. S. PEGUM
HARVEY BAKER

1

THE BIOLOGY OF THE SKIN

The skin is a frontier and protects the body against losses and incursions. It prevents the loss of water, electrolytes, proteins and other substances and thereby assists in keeping the internal environment constant; likewise, it prevents potentially dangerous micro-organisms and other foreign substances, be they solid, liquid or gaseous, entering the body. Light too is screened by the horny layer and absorbed by *melanin* pigment. With regard to radioactivity it is a complete barrier only against alpha particles. The skin protects against mechanical injury by the toughness and plasticity of the *stratum corneum* (horny layer) and by the resilient strength of the collagen and elastin of the dermis. Bacterial proliferation on the skin surface is discouraged by its dryness and a certain degree of chemical activity. Micro-organisms are actively dislodged by the constant shedding of the horny layer. The dry surface also restricts electrical conductivity by virtue of its high impedance.

In appropriate circumstances the skin may contribute vitamin D to the body's economy since dietary sterols are converted by sunlight into the vitamin. The skin is a sense organ because it is liberally endowed with sensory nerve endings sensitive to heat, cold, pain, itching and touch. It also plays a crucial role in thermal regulation; heat is conserved by contraction of the blood vessels and dissipated by the dilatation of vessels and by the secretion and evaporation of sweat.

The appendages have lost a good deal of their importance. The nails are small in man but highly developed in other animals as claws. They function as tools to pick up and manipulate fine objects. The hair has an important heat-conserving function in furry animals, but not in man. The hair that does remain on the scalp, however, protects against ultraviolet light, thereby lessening

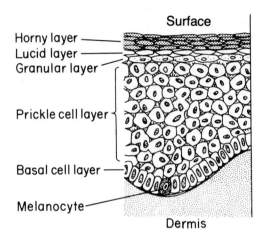

Fig. 1. Vertical section of epidermis in diagrammatic form.

the danger of solar carcinoma, and acts as a helmet against minor injury. The hair roots and the skin glands act as a source of epidermal cells for regeneration when the upper layers of the skin are destroyed.

The skin consists of the *epidermis* or outer part and the *dermis* which is beneath it (Figs 1 and 2).

THE EPIDERMIS

The epidermis has two main functions: to manufacture the barrier or horny layer of the skin, and to manufacture melanin pigment. The first task is the function of the *keratinocytes* which constitute the majority of the cell population. The second is the job of the *melanocytes*. Both cell lines are of ectodermal origin.

The basal keratinocytes of the deepest layer of the epidermis adhere by half desmosomes to the basal lamina which attaches the epidermis to the dermis. They are the parent cells of the *prickle* or *malpighian cells*, which mature as they reach the surface into non-living squames, packed with the very hard and tough protein, keratin. As the daughter cells of the basal keratinocytes move upwards they become prickle cells (Fig. 3), so called because of the appearance under the light microscope of filaments which seem to run from one cell into its neighbours. The electron microscope

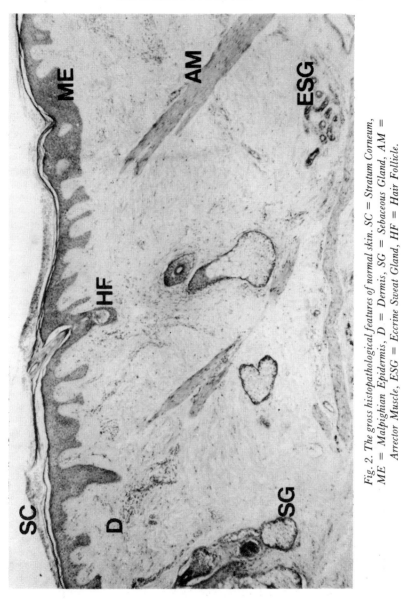

Fig. 2. The gross histopathological features of normal skin. SC = Stratum Corneum, ME = Malpighian Epidermis, D = Dermis, SG = Sebaceous Gland, AM = Arrector Muscle, ESG = Eccrine Sweat Gland, HF = Hair Follicle.

picture is different; the filaments end at the cell border in a
hemidesmosome, and the adjacent cell has a hemidesmosome in
the corresponding position. It seems as though the half desmosome
of one cell is stuck to the half desmosome of the next cell. As the
prickle cells mature they become flattened to compose the *granular
cell layer*; the granules consist of keratohyalin which is a precursor
of keratin. In some areas of epidermis, i.e. the palms and soles, the
granular layer transforms into a lucid layer, called the *stratum
lucidum*, but in most areas it matures directly into the horny layer,
or stratum corneum. The cells of the stratum corneum are composed mainly of keratin, a hard scleroprotein which contains sulphur in the form of cysteine and cystine; adjacent molecules of
cysteine combine by cross linkage, the –SH groups becoming
oxidized to –S–S– groups and making a tough bond. Horn cells
have thick cell envelopes (Fig. 4) and are tightly cemented together
by mucopolysaccharide material.

The horny layer is the barrier against penetration of the skin.
That this is so can be demonstrated in several ways. Both in vivo
and in vitro, removal of the horny layer by Sellotape stripping or
sandpapering allows vastly increased passage of all molecules

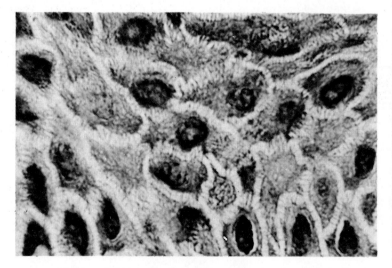

Fig. 3. Malpighian cells of the epidermis showing the 'prickles'.

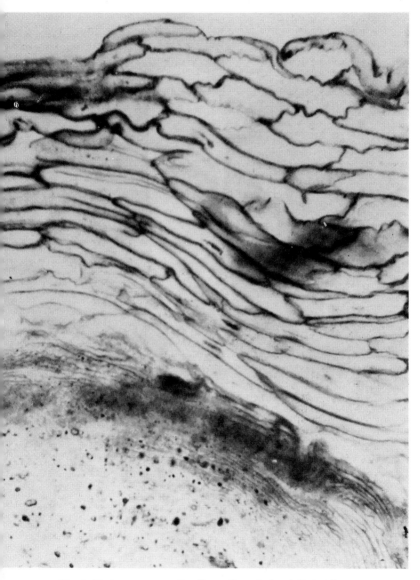

Fig. 4. Stratum corneum with cells swollen experimentally in vitro.

either way across the skin. In vivo, as the layer regenerates barrier function returns. The turnover time, i.e. the time taken for the whole epidermis to be replaced by new cells, is between 30 and 40 days, being about 14 days for the stratum corneum and 16–26 days for the viable epidermis. In certain diseases the turnover is vastly increased. Thus in psoriasis it is only about 7 days before the basal cell's daughter cell is shed from the surface as a rather immature nucleated squame. In another disease, pemphigus, the prickle cells lose their prickles (or desmosome connections) and the epidermis loses its cohesion and forms blisters.

The water holding capacity of the horny layer is of great functional importance. The cornified keratinocytes contain hygroscopic substances capable of attracting and holding water, the cell envelope acting as a semi-permeable osmotic membrane. By weight, the water content of the stratum corneum is about 10% to 15% and the ratio is critical. If the water content drops below 10%, the layer loses its plasticity and cracks allowing the entry of irritant substances, e.g. soaps. This is called chapping and it occurs if the dewpoint of the ambient air drops critically or if excessive exposure to soaps, detergents or lipid solvents has impaired the water holding capacity of the cells.

It is now realized that the essential fatty acid (EFA) component of horny layer lipids is crucial to corneal integrity. The principal fatty acids are linoleic acid of dietary origin and its derivative arachidonic acid. They are present within the lipoproteins of the cell membranes, and their unsaturated structures account for the necessary plasticity of the horny layer. EFA deficiency impairs barrier efficiency and epidermal maturation. Linoleic acid is particularly important in the 'water barrier'.

The pigment-forming cells are called *melanocytes*. Like the keratinocytes, they are of ectodermal origin, but are embryologically derived from the neural crest. During embryonic life they migrate into the epidermis and plug themselves into the basal cell layer all over the body surface. Here they are to be seen in haematoxylin and eosin stained sections as 'clear cells' with an unstained clear zone around the nucleus. Fontana or dopa stains, however, show them as dendritic cells, like nerve cells to which they are related (Fig. 5). The dendritic processes are attached to neighbouring prickle cells, into which they feed the melanosomes, the sub-cellular organelles which contain melanin.

Melanin is a brown and yellow pigment made from tyrosine under the influence of tyrosinase and conjugated with a protein. In the genetic abnormality, albinism, the melanocytes fail to produce pigment. As the keratinocytes mature into corneal cells, they take with them a complement of melanin granules which have a vital role in screening ultraviolet light, greatly reducing the amount of such light which reaches the deeper epidermis and dermis.

The third cell line making up the epidermal population is the *Langerhans' cell*. This is a dendritic cell found at higher levels in the malpighian layer. It does not synthesize melanin and is now thought to be of mesodermal origin. It was recognized a century ago by Langerhans by gold staining. Now it can easily be distinguished in electron microscope preparations by its characteristic nucleus and 'tennis racquet' organelles. There is increasing evidence that it has an immunological role, e.g. in allergic contact dermatitis.

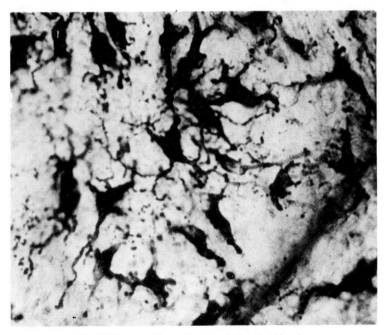

Fig. 5. Dopa-positive melanocytes in basal epidermis.

Finally, in the epidermis are also fine nerve fibres ending in Merckel's discs. Blood vessels do not penetrate into the normal epidermis.

THE DERMIS

Below the epidermis is the dermis or corium. The dermis is thicker than the epidermis and is made of connective tissue. It may be likened to a foundation garment and it keeps the soft tissues in shape. Inside the connective tissue framework are blood and lymphatic vessels, nerves, glands and a variety of cells (Fig. 2).

Connective tissue

The connective tissue is made of collagen, elastin, reticulin and ground substance. Of these collagen is the largest ingredient, accounting for 75% of the dry weight. The fibrous protein molecules have a triple helix structure and form long fibrils which show transverse striations under the electron microscope. Chemically the main amino acid constituents are glycine, proline, aniline and hydroxyproline. Collagen is also found in tendons and other body structures.

The protein elastin accounts for only a small proportion of the connective tissue. It contains the amino acid desmosine which may be responsible for the elastic properties of elastin.

Reticulin is another type of fibre which has the property of taking up silver stains.

The ground substance is mucopolysaccharide material, mainly hyaluronic acid and dermatan sulphate (chondroitin sulphate B).

Blood vessels

The circulation in the dermis nourishes the skin and its appendages and cools the body. There are three arterial plexuses, one deep at the fascial level, one between the hypoderm and the dermis and one just below the *papillae*, finger-like processes of dermis which protrude into the epidermis. The arteries empty into arterioles which are the smallest vessels to have a contractile muscular wall. The arterioles discharge into the small thin-walled capillaries which are sufficiently permeable to allow metabolites to enter and leave the adjacent tissues which they serve. Thus the nutrition of the actively metabolizing epidermis is entirely dependent on the papillary capillaries, which drain into venous plexuses.

Especially in the hands and feet, the arterioles have a certain natural, positive tone. In addition there are sympathetic fibres which produce vasoconstriction or vasodilation. Circulating or locally produced chemical mediators and metabolites can alter the arteriole tone; adrenalin and pitressin are vasoconstrictors, histamine, kinins and acetyl choline vasodilators. Local heating produces vasodilation and cooling produces vasoconstriction. Trauma of mild degree elicits the triple response of Lewis: a red line due to release of histamine which produces arteriolar dilatation in the area of injury; slightly later, another area of erythema in the surrounding skin is produced by axon reflex dilatation, dependent on the integrity of the local nerves; and, thirdly a weal is produced which is the result of fluid passing through the capillaries in the red line area where histamine has been released. An additional mechanism is also available, the glomus or arterio-venous shunt. When the powerful shunt muscle is relaxed blood can pass from the arterial to the venous side without entering the capillary network; this conserves heat. There are lymph spaces at the tip of each papilla and lymph circulates between the connective tissue fibres. Lymph channels also accompany the blood vessels.

Nerves

Both myelinated and non-myelinated sensory nerves are found in the skin. The interweaving sub-epidermal nerve nets of unmyelinated fibres have beaded terminals both in the epidermis and in the dermis. Merckel's discs are found in both situations. Three other specialized nerve endings are also found in the dermis: the Pacinian corpuscles, Krause's end bulbs and Ruffini's endings. These were thought to respond specifically to particular sensations such as pressure, cold, heat etc., but modern work has thrown doubt on this view.

Besides heat, cold, pain and light touch, itching must be regarded as a specific sensation, and not, as hitherto, as a variant of pain. Certain endopeptidases having activities in the physiological pH range will produce itching when introduced into the skin, though possibly their chief site of action is in the epidermis. Trypsin and pancreatin are examples of these substances, but others may be obtained from vegetable sources (e.g. mucunain) or from fungi (e.g. fungal proteinase). The itching experienced in maladies such as eczema may be due to accumulation or release of endopeptidases derived either from the epidermal cells or from the circulating proteolytic enzymes of the blood. Histamine and acetylcholine can each produce pruritus, but it is not known with certainty whether they are responsible for the itching which occurs in urticaria.

There are also a variety of other cells in the dermis. Fibroblasts are present in considerable number and are almost certainly responsible for making the extracellular structural materials, collagen, elastin and ground substance. The mast cells found in the vicinity of blood vessels and hair follicles contain granules which can liberate histamine and heparin, and in some animals serotonin as well.

Histiocytes, monocytes, lymphocytes and polymorphs are also found in the dermis. They are concerned with the cellular and immunological defence of the body.

Sweat glands

Sweat glands have a glomerulus or secreting part and a duct. The glomerulus consists of a coiled tube formed by a single layer of columnar cells. These are surrounded by a layer of smooth muscle, and supported by a thin fibrous capsule. Sweat glands have a relatively copious blood supply. In the dermis the duct is lined by two or three layers of cells, and pursues a straight course to the epidermis, which it enters in an interpapillary projection. Here it winds in a corkscrew fashion and opens onto the surface of the horny layer. The gland and its duct are formed by downgrowths of the epidermis.

Perspiration, both sensible and insensible, is said to represent 25% (600 ml) of the total water loss from the body in twenty-four hours under ordinary sedentary conditions. About 80% of insensible water loss is due to evaporation of small drops of sweat from the sweat duct orifices. In addition to this there is also a loss from the epidermis itself by transepidermal diffusion of perhaps 50–75 ml per day.

Sweat is a slightly turbid, almost colourless fluid, containing some 99% water. It contains small quantities of chlorides, urea, ammonia, uric acid, creatinine, phosphates, lactic acid, sulphates, certain enzymes, small amounts of the fatty acids up to caprylic, and perhaps lipoids. Sweating is under the control of the sympathetic nervous system. Acetylcholine is thought to be the chemical mediator of the nerve–sweat gland impulses.

In the genital and anal regions, the axillae, the nipples and areolae a special variety of sweat gland is found. This is an apocrine type of gland in which the tips of the cells lining the glands disintegrate and mix with the fluid secretion. The apocrine sweat glands are larger than the common, eccrine, sweat glands and many open into the hair follicles above the sebaceous glands. Their secretion is odourless until it has been contaminated with bacteria, usually micrococci, when it develops a characteristic smell (varying from race to race) which acquires a sexual significance.

OTHER FEATURES OF THE SKIN

Hypoderm

This is a transitional zone between the skin and the underlying adipose tissue. The hypoderm contains fat cells and white and yellow connective tissue. The coils of some of the sweat glands and the roots of some of the hairs are situated in the hypoderm.

Hair

The hair is epithelial in origin. It is made of modified horny cells, which arise in a follicle formed of invaginated epidermal cells situated in the deeper layers of the dermis. The follicle is a complicated structure which is itself invaginated by a small projection derived from the dermis known as the *papilla*.

The hair is formed by the proliferation of cells of the hair *matrix*, which is a layer of epidermal cells covering the underlying papilla. It is composed of three layers:
1. *The cuticle*: a thin layer of flattened horny cells.
2. *The cortex*: a thick pigmented layer of spindle-shaped cells.
3. *The medulla*: a column of cells which are nucleated near the papilla and lose their nuclei as they become more distant from it. The medulla extends for a variable distance up the hair shaft. Lanugo hairs have no medulla.

In each follicle there is a cycle of alternating phases of growth (anagen) and rest (telogen) (Fig. 6). On the human scalp, the anagen phase lasts for 2–5 years. This is followed by a resting period known as the telogen phase when there is no growth and which lasts about three months. During the telogen phase, the hair separates from its firm attachment to the papilla at the bottom of the follicle, its root becomes swollen like a club, and although it is

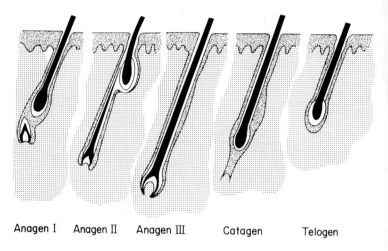

Anagen I   Anagen II   Anagen III   Catagen   Telogen

Fig. 6. The hair follicle cycle.

dead it remains in the follicle. When activity is resumed, a new hair
is formed and pushes out the old dead 'club hair' (Fig. 7). The
duration of the cycle is extremely variable but is longer in the scalp
and beard than elsewhere.

The hair cycle may be arrested if the body is subjected to insults,
such as high fever, loss of blood or a major operation. When this
happens all or nearly all the scalp hair follicles go into the resting
(telogen) phase. Two to four months after the insult a new cycle
begins and new anagen hairs displace the resting hairs. This
results in the shedding of a large amount of hair (telogen
defluvium). As a rule recovery is complete. An analogous process
but with a different mechanism may produce post partum
defluvium.

There are melanocytes in the lower portions of the hair follicles.

A small band of unstriped muscle fibres is attached to the follicle
and forms the *arrector pili* muscle. This muscle is responsible for
altering the angle at which the hair lays, e.g. when the ambient
temperature is low.

Glands

As each hair passes through the superficial layer of the dermis it is
lubricated by *sebum*, which is the excretion of a small saccular

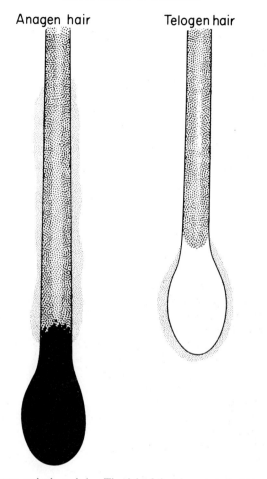

Anagen hair   Telogen hair

Fig. 7. Anagen and telogen hairs. The club of the telogen hair is depigmented.

gland formed from the epidermis. The gland lies adjacent to the hair shaft, and consists of one or several saccules with a duct which opens into the neck of the hair follicle. Sebum is formed by the fatty degeneration and disintegration of large, nucleated, polygonal cells within the gland. Human sebum is a mixture of fats and waxes. It contains free fatty acids, glycerides, esters of the higher aliphatic alcohols and cholesterol (waxes), and hydrocarbons, including squalene; its function is to lubricate the skin, keep it supple, and to protect it from becoming sodden when immersed in water, or cracked when exposed to a dry atmosphere. After puberty it has certain fungicidal properties.

Besides the sebaceous glands which are associated with hair follicles, there are others which discharge directly on to the skin surface and which are associated with the lanugo hairs. The Meibomian glands on the eyelids and Tyson's glands on the *glans penis* and inner surface of the prepuce are modified, large sebaceous glands. The glands of the mucous surfaces of the lips, the areolae and the genitalia are also modified sebaceous glands.

Nails

The nails consist of modified horny cells firmly united. They are formed proximally in the nail matrix, which consists of modified cells from the Malpighian layer. The nail bed, which underlies the main mass of the nail, consists of somewhat modified prickle cells,

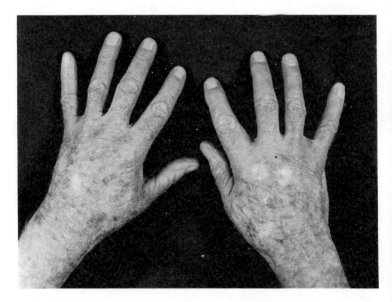

Fig. 8. Solar damage to the skin on the back of the hand.

to which the nail is firmly attached. The papillae in the dermis underlying the nail bed are arranged to form a series of longitudinal ridges. As a very rough estimate, it may be said that a fingernail takes from five to six months to grow from the matrix to the finger tip; but there are seasonal variations in the rate of growth. The toenails take at least twice as long to grow.

THE EFFECTS OF LIGHT ON THE SKIN

The sun's radiation, particularly the ultra-violet band between 295 and 400nm wavelength, is the principal factor responsible for normal ageing of skin. Its effects are directly proportional to the amount of melanin protection, which is genetically determined, and the cumulative amount of ultra-violet exposure. Actinic damage affects both the epidermis and dermis and is seen mainly on the head and neck, backs of hands (Fig. 8) and forearms. In the epidermis, thinning, hyperpigmentation (solar lentigo), depigmentation and dyskeratosis (solar keratosis) are seen. Solar keratosis may develop into frank carcinoma. In the dermis, collagen and elastic degradation decrease the bulk of the skin making it thin and wrinkled. The unsupported dermal blood vessels bleed easily on minor trauma, e.g. senile purpura.

2

THE PRINCIPLES OF DIAGNOSIS

As in every branch of medicine, diagnosis is based on history and examination. However, skin diseases can often be recognized at a glance, so a brief, preliminary look at the skin can save time in history taking.

THE HISTORY

The following questions are important when investigating the history of a particular instance of skin disease. When and where did the trouble start? How did it spread? Has its subsequent course been phasic or continuous? Does it itch? Does it 'weep'? Have the mouth, the scalp or the nails been involved? Has the patient noticed any provocative factors? If chronic over years, is it seasonal?

Any treatment, either internal or external, that could possibly be related to the disorder must be documented. What drugs was the patient taking, for any reason, prior to, subsequent to or at the time of onset? What local treatments have been applied to the affected skin, both prescribed and otherwise? Have any of the applications patently aggravated the rash? Often it is necessary to make specific enquiries about steroids, antibiotics, antiseptics, etc.

The patient's environment must also be investigated. What is his occupation? What are his hobbies? What chemical exposures are known at work or at leisure? Does the rash improve at weekends and worsen from Monday to Friday? Has it cleared up during annual holidays or periods off work? What is the effect of sunlight?

Finally, enquiry into previous illnesses, family history and any symptoms in sexual or social contacts must never be neglected.

THE EXAMINATION

Certain principles are of prime importance when examining the skin. 'Peep-hole' diagnosis should be avoided. Examine the whole organ. If the patient is not undressed, relevant lesions can be missed. Thus, an elderly patient with widespread eczema may have a chronic leg ulcer to which a sensitizer is being applied; the patient may regard this as irrelevant and not mention it. Never examine an eruption of the hands and neglect to look at the feet. In a baby always examine the napkin area.

A good light is essential for the examination, and natural light is

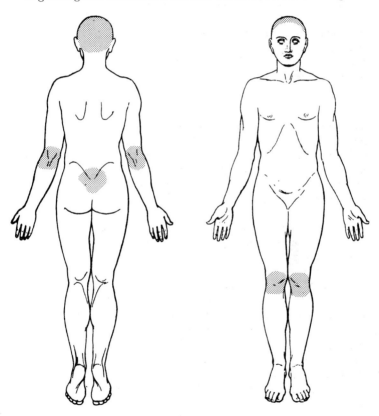

Fig. 9. Psoriasis: distribution of lesions.

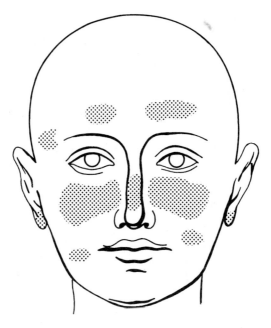

Fig. 10. Lupus erythematosus: distribution of lesions.

ideal. The burrows of scabies can easily be missed in poor light. When the patient is ready, look at the overall distribution of the eruption before studying the morphological details. The distribution of the rash can point strongly to the diagnosis even before its morphology has been considered. Certain diseases such as psoriasis, scabies, acne, lichen planus, seborrhoeic eczema, pityriasis rosea, atopic eczema and lupus erythematosus have a very characteristic pattern (see Figs 9 to 16). Is the eruption symmetrical or asymmetrical? Is it centrifugal or centripetal? Does it have a predilection for extensor or flexor surfaces? Is it confined to light-exposed areas?

A rapid inspection will determine if the eruption is monomorphic or polymorphic. In polymorphic eruptions each of the different types of lesions must be carefully studied in turn. Finally, never neglect to look carefully at the nails, the hair and the mouth, or to make any obviously relevant further examination, e.g. palpa-

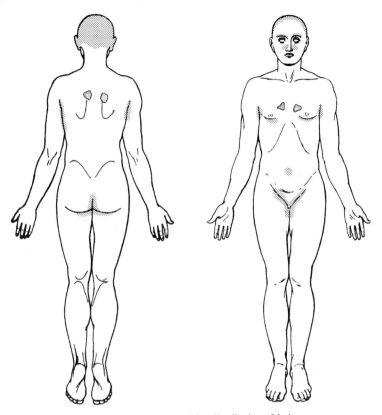

Fig. 11. Seborrhoeic dermatitis: distribution of lesions.

tion of lymph glands in the differential diagnosis of a neoplasm or palpation of peripheral arterial pulses where ischaemia is suspected. It should also be mentioned that palpation of skin lesions themselves is vital. Both the eyes and the finger tips are needed for dermatological diagnosis.

TERMINOLOGY

It is impossible to succinctly record or describe an eruption without the use of terms with an accepted conventional meaning. The following are used.

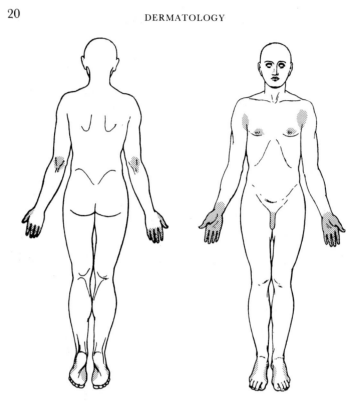

Fig. 12. Scabetic burrows: distribution of lesions.

PRIMARY LESIONS

Macules

Macules are areas of discoloration of the skin. They are visible but not palpable, being neither raised nor depressed nor thickened. They may be of any size. Macules may be erythematous, purpuric, pigmented or depigmented.

Papules

Papules are palpable elevations of the skin varying from about 1–5 mm in diameter. Their surfaces may be pointed, rounded or flat.

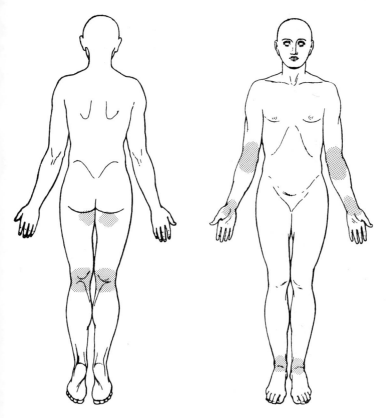

Fig. 13. Atopic eczema: distribution of lesions.

They are not deep seated in the skin, and are formed by proliferation of the cells, or by exudation of fluids into the skin. The typical lesions of lichen planus and acne are papules.

Nodules

Nodules are larger than papules, and they may be more deeply seated in the skin. Lesions in the subcutaneous tissues may form nodules, e.g. the nodules of rheumatoid arthritis. Nodules may be hard like carcinomatous secondary deposits or soft as in Von Recklinghausen's neurofibromatosis.

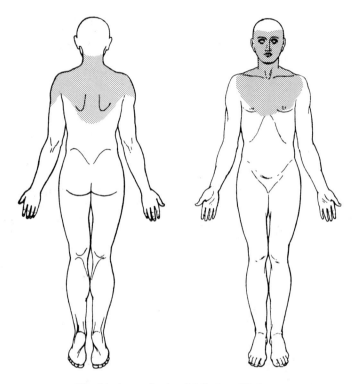

Fig. 14. Acne vulgaris: distribution of lesions.

Vesicles

Vesicles are small blisters formed by the accumulation of fluid in the skin and associated with the disintegration of the cells of the affected areas. They are usually filled with serous fluid.

Bullae

Bullae are large blisters. They are uni-locular or multi-locular, and may be of enormous size. They may be intra-epidermal or sub-epidermal. Bullae may contain serum, sero-purulent or haemorrhagic fluid.

Pustules

A pustule is a vesicle containing pus, i.e. it is packed with polymor-

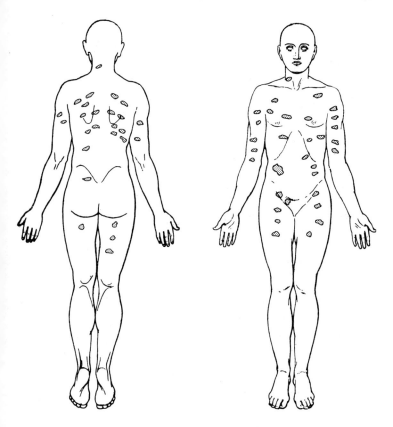

Fig. 15. Pityriasis rosea: distribution of lesions.

phonuclear leucocytes and serum. It should be noted that pustulosis may be non-infective, as in acne vulgaris or pustular psoriasis. Pustules may arise on ordinary skin or may be follicular in origin.

Erythema

Erythema is redness of the skin caused by vascular dilatation. It may be transient or chronic. Erythema can be blanched. Various shades and hues of erythema are seen in various diseases.

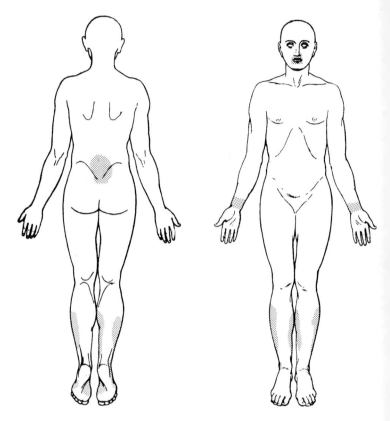

Fig. 16. Lichen planus: distribution of lesions.

Purpura

Purpura is extravasation of blood into the skin. Purpura does not blanch. The blood in the tissue is degraded within phagocytes to haemosiderin which is a brown pigment. Chronic purpura, e.g. from capillaritis, may produce a golden rash, the colour being due to the admixture of old and new purpura.

Weals

Weals are elevations of the skin caused by oedema of the dermis.

They are sometimes linear in shape and are usually erythematous. Weals are caused by an increased permeability of the walls of the blood capillaries.

Scales

Scales indicate an abnormality of the process of keratinization of the epidermal cells, and are found when imperfectly keratinized cells of the horny layer (which may be nucleated) adhere together. They may be small, as in dandruff, or large, as in psoriasis.

Burrows

Burrows are irregular, short, linear elevations of the horny layer, and are usually dark or speckled black. They are the characteristic lesions of scabies.

Blackheads

Blackheads are small plugs of laminated horny cells and sebum blocking the pilo-sebaceous orifices. They are the primary lesions of acne vulgaris.

Plaques

Plaques are circumscribed flat areas of abnormal skin or mucous membrane, which may be raised above or sunk below the level of the surrounding skin. Examples are the plaques of scleroderma or leucoplakia.

Benign or malignant tumours and cysts may also develop in the skin (see Chapter 22).

SECONDARY LESIONS

Fissures

Fissures are small cracks extending through the epidermis so that the dermis is exposed.

Ulcers

Ulcers are lesions formed by destruction of the whole skin, e.g. by ischaemia, infection or neoplasia. The base of an ulcer may be granulation tissue, tendon, etc. but cannot be any layer of the skin.

Erosion

Erosion is a more superficial loss of tissue whose base is in the skin. Thus, the whole epidermis may be eroded leaving a lesion whose base is the dermis or erosions can be very superficial, only part of the epidermis being lost as in pemphigus.

Atrophy

Atrophy implies shrinkage of skin. The epidermis may be atrophic, as in ischaemic skin, or the dermis may become atrophic due to loss of collagen, e.g. from life-long exposure to sunlight.

Hypertrophy

Hypertrophy is a meaningless term unless the site of tissue overgrowth is specified. Thus, epidermal hypertrophy (increased volume) may be due to acanthosis in which the Malpighian layer is expanded, hyperkeratosis in which the stratum corneum is thickened but otherwise fairly normal or parakeratosis in which a thickened loose scaly stratum corneum is quantitatively and qualitatively deranged. Dermal hypertrophy may consist of collagen, as in a keloid, or consist of any other of the dermal components.

Scars

Scars develop as part of a healing process and consist of avascular connective tissue in the dermis and often sub-cutis. The epidermis over a dermal scar is usually atrophic.

Crusts

Crusts are of three varieties: red-black blood crusts; yellow-green pus crusts; and honey-coloured serum crusts.

SPECIAL INVESTIGATIONS IN DIAGNOSIS

The following simple techniques are of great value in the diagnosis of skin complaints.

Swabbing

Swabbing is a method for obtaining bacteriological or viral specimens for culture. Aspiration of fluid from an intact vesicle or pustule is usually more valuable than swabbing an open surface, although the latter may be needed e.g. in ulceration.

Scrapings of the stratum corneum

Stratum corneum scrapings are taken for microscopy and culture when investigating ringworm fungi or yeast infections. A blade moistened in 10% potassium hydroxide is used to scrape the affected surface, and the material obtained is transferred to a glass slide for direct microscopy. For culture a dry blade is used to transfer scrapings to a piece of black paper which is folded and sealed for transmission to the laboratory.

Wood's light examination

This is invaluable in the diagnosis of tinea capitis and erythrasma. (See pp. 80 and 95.)

Biopsy

When doubt exists concerning a diagnosis, there are few measures which give more assistance than microscopical examination of a well-prepared section of tissue taken from the affected zone.

The biopsy site chosen should be one where the eruption is most representative of the whole clinical picture; as far as possible, areas of secondary change should be avoided. After infiltrating the anaesthetic, an oval area of the lesions is removed with a scalpel blade, which is kept vertical to the skin surface to avoid 'shelving' the specimen. Forceps should only be applied to one end of the specimen to facilitate removal. A piece 12 mm by 4 mm usually will suffice. The wound is then closed with sutures and, if this is carefully done, scarring is negligible, especially on the face. Biopsy specimens are usually cut from the edge of an eruption because they must include the full thickness of skin and also an area of apparently normal skin.

When the specimen has been removed, it should be immediately placed on a small piece of filter-paper, and then dropped into 10 per cent formol-saline. A cylindrical biopsy specimen 3 mm to 6 mm in diameter can be obtained using a 'punch' biopsy instrument. After the cylinder of tissue is cut, it is gently lifted out with forceps and its base severed with scissors. With small punches, i.e. less than 4 mm in diameter, a stitch is unnecessary.

3

THE PRINCIPLES OF TREATMENT

Although many skin diseases are treated systemically, dermatological treatment has the additional dimension of topical therapy. Because topical therapy is so unlike the systemic administration of drugs to which the student has been introduced from his earliest clinical days, he often finds it difficult to understand. This chapter is a brief attempt to explain topical and systemic therapy on a rational basis.

TOPICAL THERAPY

THE AIMS OF TOPICAL THERAPY

Local applications may have many aims other than the exposure of the skin to specific pharmacological agents. Such aims include:

Cooling

Cooling raises the threshold of itching and so reduces pruritus.

Drying

Drying or astringency is of value in exudative conditions and reduces the risk of secondary bacterial infection of the skin surface.

Hydration

Hydrating the skin may be of value when the stratum corneum is abnormally dry as in ichthyosis or chapping. The stratum corneum is only pliable and healthy when its water content falls within a certain narrow range (see p. 6). In other circumstances, hydrating the corneum increases its permeability to pharmacological agents. This type of drug may be incorporated in an occlusive paraffin base which prevents water loss from the skin surface.

Crust removal

The removal of crusts may be important because it allows access of antibiotics to the skin below, e.g. in impetigo.

Scale removal

Removing scale has the same therapeutic value as removing crusts, but it is also of cosmetic importance and increases skin pliability and hence the patient's comfort.

Protection

Visible skin lesions attract the attention of the patient's fingers, even in the absence of pruritus. Rubbing and scratching increase skin damage, promote lichenification and encourage secondary infection. Thick pastes and ointments physically protect the skin from the fingers and hide the lesions from the eyes, lessening the urge to molest.

Drug administration

Specific drug therapy with topical anti-inflammatory agents, antibiotics, etc, brings a drug directly to the target organ where it is wanted and minimizes the exposure of other organs where it is unwanted, thus removing one of the chief drawbacks of systemic drug administration. Such treatment necessitates incorporating the active drug in a suitable vehicle or base. The vehicle must be suitably designed for the carriage and release of the drug and also be compatible with the other aims and requirements of topical therapy in each particular clinical situation.

QUALITIES AND TYPES OF VEHICLE FOR TOPICAL THERAPY

The ideal vehicle or base for topical therapy should not be irritating or sensitizing. It should not react with the stratum corneum or the active agent and should allow the release of the agent into the skin. It should be stable at room temperature, have a long shelf life and must not tolerate growth of micro-organisms within it during storage. Its colour and consistency must be physically and cosmetically acceptable to the patient.

Lotions

Lotions are liquid vehicles which may or may not be volatile. A lotion may be aqueous or alcoholic or may contain other volatile components. Evaporation of the vehicle promotes cooling and rapidly increases the concentration of active drug. Lotions with an oily base are called liniments, e.g. oily calamine lotion.

Shake lotions

Shake lotions contain an inert powder in aqueous suspension. Evaporation of the water promotes cooling and leaves a protective deposit of powder, e.g. calamine lotion.

Creams

Creams are emulsions of either water-in-oil (oily creams) or oil-in-water (vanishing creams). An emulsifying agent is needed to keep the system stable. In an emulsion the active agent is dispersed between the oil and water phases according to its partition coefficient. The advantages of such emulsions include miscibility with surface exudation, ease of removal and patient acceptability. Oil-in-water emulsions do not feel greasy and do not retard heat loss.

Ointments

Ointments may be either hydrophylic or hydrophobic. A hydrophylic ointment is miscible with water, e.g. wool alcohols (lanolin) ointment. A hydrophobic ointment is not miscible with water and is stiffer and greasy e.g. soft white paraffin (Vaseline). Hydrophobic ointments have the advantage of preventing heat loss when this is desirable and hydrating the stratum corneum. Drugs are suspended rather than dissolved in an ointment which promotes easy release of the drug into the skin.

Pastes

Pastes contain a high proportion of powder such as starch or zinc oxide in an ointment base. Pastes can be made very stiff allowing application of a drug to precisely defined lesions, e.g. the use of dithranol in psoriasis. They may also play an important protective role. Lassar's paste contains 24% of zinc oxide, 24% starch, 2% salicylic acid with 50% of soft white paraffin.

Dusting powders

Dusting powders contain zinc oxide, starch or purified talc and are useful as drying agents, absorbers of heat, or occasionally as vehicles for drugs.

Sun screens

These are useful in patients with photosensitivity. Lotions and creams are available. They screen out short-wave ultra-violet B rays more effectively than the longer ultra-violet A wavelengths. Mexenone 4% cream (Uvistat, U.K.; Solbar[R], Uval[R], U.S.A.) is useful, but lotions containing para-aminobenzoate esters are probably superior and more cosmetically effective, e.g. Spectraban Lotion, U.K.; Blockout[R], Pabafilm[R], U.S.A.

In sensitivity to UVA or visible light, preparations containing burned sugar, red veterinary petroleum jelly or titanium dioxide may be useful, e.g. Covering Cream, E. Arden, U.K.; Afil[R], Reflecta[R], U.S.A.

Soaps

Soaps have a useful defatting action in the seborrhoea of acne vulgaris. A soap medicated with an antiseptic (e.g. Cidal, U.K.; Dial[R], Palmolive Gold[R], U.S.A.) may have a place in the treatment and prevention of furunculosis. Simple Soap (U.K.) is free of perfume and other additives which may be useful in perfume-sensitive individuals.

Detergents

These are of value as shampoos. 1% cetrimide shampoo has a useful antiseptic action. Detergent shampoos, medicated with tar, have a place in the treatment of pityriasis capitis and scalp psoriasis, e.g. Polytar, U.K. & U.S.A.

Metals

Zinc oxide powder is very widely used, chiefly as an inert powder to alter the consistency of lotions, creams, pastes and ointments, much as cornflour is used to thicken gravy. Starch powder is used for a similar purpose. Calamine is basic zinc carbonate or zinc oxide coloured with ferric oxide, which avoids the striking dead white appearance of zinc oxide on the skin. Titanium dioxide is sometimes added to applications to make them more acceptable cosmetically and also acts as a sun screen. Copper and zinc sulphate lotion (B.P.C.) is a valuable after-shave lotion for those who tend to suffer from infected hair follicles on the beard area. Aluminium acetate solution (B.P.C.), sometimes called Burow's solution, 5% in water, is a mildly astringent solution used as a compress for the oozing stage of various dermatoses.

Medicated dressings

These are of several types. Salicylic acid in a concentration up to 40% may be incorporated into plasters which are cut to shape and applied to plantar warts for 24–48 hours at a time. Bland zinc ointments or ointments containing tar or iodoquinolines can be incorporated into bandages which can be left on areas of lichenified eczema for several days at a time (see p. 142). A proprietary steroid medicated, translucent, adhesive tape containing flurandrenolone (Haelan Tape, U.K.; Cordan Tape^R, U.S.A.) is useful in chronic localized inflammatory skin disease which is resistant to conventional therapy and may be used in eczema, psoriasis, lichen planus and discoid lupus erythematosus.

SPECIFIC DRUGS USED TOPICALLY

Anti-bacterial antibiotics can be used in the topical treatment of skin disease. Where time and resources permit, topical antibiotic therapy should be guided, like its systemic use, by bacteriological culture. Penicillins and streptomycin are *never* used topically because of their sensitizing potential. All those listed below are used, but they can all occasionally sensitize the skin. Neomycin is probably the most sensitizing and tetracycline the least.

Chlortetracycline

Chlortetracycline is a bacteriostatic antibiotic that is active against most strains of *Streptococcus pyogenes*, although many strains of *Staphylococcus aureus* are resistant. It also has some activity against Gram-negative organisms.

Neomycin

Neomycin is a very valuable antibiotic for topical use because it is not used systemically and is active against most strains of *Staphylococcus aureus*. It has no activity against *Streptococcus pyogenes*. When used for long periods on eczematous skin neomycin has a considerable predilection to sensitize. It should not be used on ulcers since absorption has occasionally led to nerve deafness or renal damage.

Bacitracin and gramicidin

These are two valuable antibiotics which are not used systemically. *Streptococcus pyogenes* is always sensitive to both as are some strains of *Staphylococcus aureus*. Either bacitracin or gramicidin is used in combination with neomycin. This alignment is of particular value in treating impetigo and infected eczema where both *Streptococcus pyogenes* and *Staphylococcus aureus* may be present.

Fucidic acid

This antibiotic is very active against Gram-positive cocci and has been widely used topically. Used systemically, it is a valuable agent in serious systemic staphylococcal infections such as osteomyelitis and post-influenzal pneumonia, and it is therefore the authors' belief that the topical use of fucidic acid should be restricted so as not to encourage the emergence of bacterial resistance.

Gentamicin

Gentamicin is active against *Staphylococcus aureus* and *Pseudomonas aeruginosa*. Like neomycin it is inactive against *Streptococcus pyogenes*. It is used systemically and considerations similar to those for fucidic acid apply.

Polymyxin

Polymyxin is not used systemically and has a useful range of activity against Gram-negative organisms. It is used in combination with neomycin or bacitracin.

Chloramphenicol

Chloramphenicol (Chloromycetin, U.K.) is a cheap wide-spectrum antibiotic which is active against a range of Gram-positive and Gram-negative organisms. Because its systemic use was greatly restricted 20 years ago as it may rarely cause a fatal aplastic anaemia, bacterial resistance is very uncommon. However, it can sensitize the skin to produce an allergic contact dermatitis.

Sulphonamides

Sulphonamides are not used topically on the skin because of their sensitizing potential. Sodium sulphacetamide drops (Albucid, U.K.) are used in the eye.

Antihistamines

Antihistamines should not be used topically because of their sensitizing potential. In any case they have no antihistaminic action when applied topically and allay itching by virtue of their local anaesthetic potential.

Local anaesthetics

Local anaesthetics of the procaine series (e.g. amethocaine and benzocaine) should not be used because of the risk of sensitization. Lignocaine (Xylocaine, U.K.) virtually never sensitizes and has a limited role in ano-genital pruritus.

Antiseptics

Potassium permanganate is an extremely useful non-sensitizing astringent and wide-spectrum antiseptic. It is used in a dilute aqueous solution of between 1:4000 and 1:16 000 for a few minutes daily as a wet compress or by immersion of the affected part. Other antiseptics include benzalkonium chloride 0.1% and chlorhexidine gluconate 1% (Hibitane, U.K.). Iodoquinolines (Chinoform, Clioquinol, Chlorquinaldol) are useful wide-spectrum agents but occasionally sensitize.

Anti-fungal agents

Basic dyes such as 1% aqueous gentian violet lotion are highly effective against fungal infections but tend to be messy and ruin linen. Potassium permanganate and iodoquinolines are very useful. Antibiotics active against *Candida albicans* include nystatin and amphotericin B. Clotrimazole and miconazole nitrate are of particular value, being active against dermatophytes, *Candida* species, tinea versicolor and some bacteria. Griseofulvin is not active topically.

SYSTEMIC THERAPY

The principles of systemic therapy for skin disease do not differ from those appropriate for any other disease. Systemic therapy has a limited usefulness and is usually used in conjunction with topical therapy.

Analgesics

Itching is generally more important than pain and it is rarely necessary to use analgesics stronger than aspirin or paracetamol.

Anti-pruritic agents

Antihistamines are the principal drugs used for pruritus. There is a wide range with varying sedative side-effects. These side-effects may be useful, especially at night, but drivers or those handling machinery should be particularly warned about the sedative actions. Sedatives such as diazepam and nitrazepam may also be useful in allaying itching.

Non-steroid anti-inflammatory agents

Indomethacin (Indocid, U.K.) and phenylbutazone (Butazolidin, U.K.) may have a place in cutaneous vascular disease including superficial thrombophlebitis and nodular vasculitis.

Corticosteroids

These suppress but never cure disease. Their disadvantages include a lowering of resistance to many infections, metabolic disturbances (particularly in regard to electrolytes and carbohydrates leading to fluid retention), oedema (moon face, buffalo hump), increase in weight, a steady increase in diastolic blood pressure (often in systolic pressure too), osteoporosis, emotional disturbances, and the appearance of hirsuties, acne and striae (Fig. 17). Obviously patients must be carefully selected for corticosteroid treatment and as carefully supervised when under treatment. The minimum care demands an initial X-ray of the chest to exclude pulmonary tuberculosis, regular recordings of weight and blood-pressure, and regular examinations for glycosuria; these should be done at least once a month in ambulant cases. Estimations of serum electrolyte levels are made if oedema is

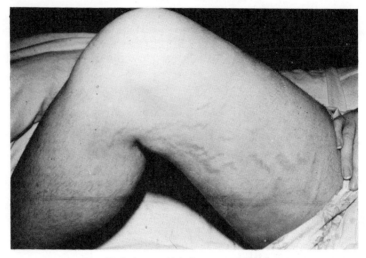

Fig. 17. Striae on thigh due to steroid therapy.

troublesome. Also, a matter which is too often omitted, X-ray investigation of at least part of the thoracic spine should be undertaken from time to time to ensure that osteoporosis is not occurring. Deviations from the normal in any of these investigations demand careful attention and appropriate action on the part of the physician. Sometimes iatrogenic abnormalities discovered by these tests necessitate abandoning steroid therapy. Patients must be warned never suddenly to stop taking steroids, for intense fatigue, prostration, and even collapse from adrenal insufficiency are likely unless they are weaned slowly. Patients must also be told that, should they have to have an anaesthetic, even 'gas' for the removal of a tooth, they must warn the anaesthetist, and this caveat must be remembered for two years after ceasing to take the drug. The patient should carry a steroid record card.

Prednisolone is the drug usually used. Initial dosage depends on the disease being treated. It may be quite small (10 – 15 mg daily) in a chronic eczema, rather higher in very acute urticaria, contact dermatitis or pompholyx eczema (30 – 40 mg daily) and still higher in dermatomyositis, systemic lupus erythematosus or bullous pemphigoid (50 – 60 mg daily). Even higher doses, up to 360 mg daily, may be needed for short periods in pemphigus vulgaris.

The dose is reduced as soon as the disease comes under control. Where maintenance therapy is necessary, the smallest possible dosage should always be used. There is some evidence that alternate day therapy is a safer schedule for long-term treatment.

Corticotrophin has been largely superseded by its synthetic analogue, tetracosactrin zinc (Synacthen Depot, U.K.). Both have the disadvantage of having to be given by injection. They also have a greater sodium retaining potential than prednisolone.

Antibiotics

Only a few antibiotics have a regular place in therapy. Penicillin (benzylpenicillin or phenoxymethylpenicillin) is the treatment of choice in erysipelas and secondary streptococcal infections (e.g. in eczema). If the patient is allergic to penicillin, erythromycin is the second choice. Erythromycin and flucloxacillin are the two main anti-staphylococcal antibiotics and only rarely will fucidic acid, gentamicin or clindamycin be needed for such infections. Ampicillin and its derivatives have virtually no place in skin therapy. Co-trimoxazole is sometimes useful for Gram-positive coccal infection. In long term prophylaxis after recurrent bouts of erysipelas, sulphadimidine can be considered as an alternative to penicillin or erythromycin. The sulphone, dapsone, is used only in the treatment of leprosy and (not as an antibiotic) in dermatitis herpetiformis (see p. 177). Griseofulvin is an antibiotic specifically active against the dermatophytes which cause tinea, but is of no value in candidosis or tinea versicolor.

Vitamins

Vitamin A is known to influence keratinization and large doses are sometimes used in certain rare disorders of keratinization. In the absence of vitamin deficiency, there is no evidence that vitamins have any value in the treatment of skin disease.

Iron

In rare cases, iron deficiency is a cause of alopecia which can be corrected by oral iron therapy.

PHYSICAL THERAPY

Ultra-violet light

Short wave ultra-violet (UVB) irradiation is of value in psoriasis and acne vulgaris. Long wave irradiation (UVA) is used in the management of psoriasis and, to a lesser extent, in vitiligo in conjunction with the photo-active drug, 8-methoxypsoralen.

X-rays

Irradiation with X-rays has an established place in the treatment of malignant skin disease. Squamous and basal cell carcinomata are often treated by radiotherapy as an alternative to surgical extirpation. X-rays are of little value in malignant melonoma. Radiation may be of value in cutaneous lymphoma, e.g. mycosis fungoides, when whole body electron beam therapy is sometimes used.

Radiotherapy is now little used for benign skin disease but low voltage 10 kV (Grenz) irradiation may have a small place in the management of chronic eczema. X-ray epilation for tinea capitis was abandoned when the antibiotic griseofulvin became available.

The effects of X-rays on normal skin depend on dosage and the elapse of time. Mild chronic radiodermatitis consists of atrophy, telangiectasia and pigmentary disturbance. In more severe damage radio-necrotic ulceration may be caused. There is a long-term carcinogenic hazard, evident 15 – 50 years after exposure.

Cryotherapy

The application of extreme cold to living tissue leads to irreversible damage and cell death. Liquefied nitrogen is used for this purpose and is a convenient, safe and easily controllable form of treatment. The liquid nitrogen can be applied simply and accurately by means of an orange stick-mounted cotton wool bud, a method which suffices for most simple work. Various forms of apparatus are available which are needed for tumour treatment. Cryotherapy is of value in the treatment of viral warts, basal cell papilloma (seborrhoeic wart) and skin tags.

Dermabrasion

Dermabrasion is a surgical technique, sometimes called skin planing. The patient is made relaxed and drowsy with suitable sedatives or given a general anaesthetic, and the eyes and lips are carefully shielded with special guards. Using a proper aseptic technique a small area of skin is frozen by spraying with a suitable volatile liquid, e.g. a mixture of freons with or without ethyl chloride. When solid, the skin surface is abraded to a suitable depth by a rapidly revolving wire brush or burr, mounted on an apparatus similar to a dentist's drill. Adjacent areas of skin are then rapidly frozen and dealt with, and any bleeding is controlled by pressure. Non-adhering types of dressings are then applied. The abraded surface heals within ten days leaving the skin somewhat pink. Later, milia may appear in the treated area and have to be removed. The operation is especially successful on the face, but less successful elsewhere. There is less risk of abnormal scarring in white than in pigmented skins. Dermabrasion is chiefly used to lessen the unsightliness of depressed scars, especially those which develop in acne vulgaris.

Diathermy

Fulguration and coagulation with electric currents are used in dermatology; the cutting current is also employed. By a special technique permanent epilation of hirsute areas can be undertaken with diathermy, without leaving scars.

Electrocautery

This is a very valuable technique for destroying small lesions. It is also used after curettage to stop bleeding and to destroy wart virus.

Electrolysis

A direct current of 1 – 2 milliamperes is required for electrolysis. The positive lead is attached to an indifferent electrode and the negative to a needle-holder bearing a very fine platinum-iridium needle or a steel needle of size 12. A switch is incorporated in the needle-holder. Electrolysis is used to permanently remove superfluous hair and small capillary naevi. In epilation the needle is passed down the hair follicle, and the current allowed to flow for about 20 seconds, when small bubbles of hydrogen appear at the orifice of the follicle. The hair loosens and may be removed without tugging.

A small dilated blood vessel may be occluded by threading the needle down its lumen and passing a current for 15 – 30 seconds.

4

GENETIC DISORDERS OF THE SKIN

Genetic disorders are conditions which are transmitted from parents to their offspring by the chromosomes. The inheritance may be dominant, recessive or sex-linked recessive. Tuberose sclerosis and neurofibromatosis, both fibrous dysplasias involving the skin and the nervous system, ichthyosis vulgaris and hereditary haemorrhagic telangiectasia are examples of dominant inheritance, while total albinism and phenylketonuria are recessive. A special type of ichthyosis is sex-linked and affects males only. Male type baldness is of dominant transmission but only shows itself in the male when circulating androgen appears at puberty, hence it is sex-limited. In a number of other diseases, such as psoriasis, alopecia areata, vitiligo and atopic dermatitis, inheritance plays an important role but environmental factors may be required to trigger an actual attack.

Ichthyosis

Ichthyosis, or fish skin disease, is characterized by dry scaly skin (Fig. 18). The basic defect is probably an inability to form a normal horny layer so that there is an increased water permeability and the horny cells themselves are unable to hold water and remain inadequately hydrated. The lipid metabolism of the epidermis may be abnormal because scaly skin is a feature of induced or inherited inhibition of lipid synthesis.

Ichthyosis vulgaris is the commonest variety and is inherited as an autosomal dominant. Dryness and scaling begin in the first few months of life. The scales are whitish or brown in colour and affect the arms, legs and trunk. The axillae, the popliteal and antecubital fossae are usually normal. Scaling of the forehead and cheeks is seen in children but clears as they get older. The knees, elbows and ankles are often hyperkeratotic. Follicular keratosis (keratosis

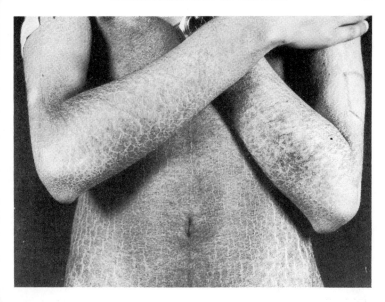

Fig. 18. Ichthyosis.

pilaris) may be present. The palms and soles show an exaggeration of the normal creases.

Other types of ichthyosis include: a mild xeroderma, frequently found in those with atopic eczema; X-linked ichthyosis, a severe form which affects males and produces larger scales, often yellow-brown or even black; and, follicular ichthyosis. Some ichthyoses are most severe at birth, for example the 'Collodion baby' syndrome may clear completely or continue as ichthyosiform erythrodermia, depending on genetic factors. A very severe type, the Harlequin fetus, may be lethal.

Treatment. The skin should be hydrated by bathing and cleaned with aqueous cream (B.P.) or emulsifying ointment (B.P.) in place of soap. Excess scales can be removed by scrubbing or by pumice stone. Soft paraffin (petrolatum), emulsifying ointment or a 10% urea cream (Calmurid, U.K.) is applied. Ichthyosis improves in a warm fairly humid atmosphere and becomes worse in a cold climate, when fissuring and eczematization can develop. Ichthyosis vulgaris tends to improve with age.

NEUROFIBROMATOSIS

Neurofibromatosis or von Recklinghausen's Disease is usually dominantly inherited but variable in its clinical expression. The first signs in childhood are often axillary 'freckling' and the development of *café au lait* spots (see Fig. 95). Six or more *café au lait* spots of a diameter greater than 2.5 cm are said to be diagnostic. Later, perhaps in the teens or in early adult life, the nodules or tumours (molluscum fibrosum) develop in the dermis from the Schwann cells of the peripheral nerves (Fig. 19). They are soft and pink or bluish and can number from a few to hundreds. They may spread along a nerve forming plexiform neuroma or produce elephantiasis neuromatosa. Kyphosis, scoliosis and other bony changes occur. Oligophrenia is frequent. Tumours may affect the optic, auditory and spinal nerves and produce compression. Intra-cranial tumours may cause epilepsy. Sarcomatous changes can occur.

Treatment. The nodules and tumours may be removed, but in severe cases the large number of lesions can make this a daunting task.

TUBEROSE SCLEROSIS

Tuberose sclerosis (epiloia, Bourneville's disease, adenoma sebaceum) is of autosomal dominant inheritance and is characterized by fibromata or angiofibromata in various organs. An infant suffering 'jack knife' fits or other neurological disturbance should be closely examined for small white ash-leaf areas of leukoderma which are often the first skin sign. The use of Wood's light in a dark room may be helpful in this examination. In childhood or later, skin coloured or pink papules with telangiectasia appear on the cheeks and nose in a 'muzzle' distribution. Although these papules are called adenoma sebaceum, they are really angiofibromas. Fibromata of the nail folds and shagreen patches of the skin are also seen.

The lesions in the CNS produce mental deficiency, secondary dementia and epilepsy. The eyes, lungs, heart and kidneys may also be affected.

XANTHOMATOSIS

Yellow or orange lesions in the skin which are due to deposition of lipids are called xanthomata. Sebaceous naevi may have a similar colour. Xanthelasma is a flat or slightly raised xanthomatosis of the eyelids; it is common and the blood lipids may be normal or

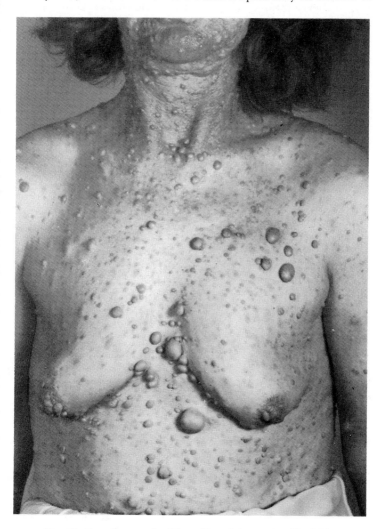

Fig. 19. Neurofibromatosis. (For café au lait *spots see Fig. 95.)*

abnormal. Tuberous xanthomas are soft, painless plaques, papules or tumours over the elbows, buttocks or knees, and are associated with hyperlipoproteinaemia (Plate I). Eruptive xanthomas develop rapidly in showers, on the elbows, buttocks and back. They may be fiery red and angry or itching at first. They indicate an increase in the serum triglycerides. Tendon xanthomas are swellings which may be tender or even painful in the Achilles tendon or tendons of the hands and feet. They are usually associated with lipid abnormality of Type IIa (see below). Plane xanthomas are flat or slightly elevated with abnormal or normal serum lipid levels and are in some cases associated with dysglobulinaemia, myeloma or lymphoma.

Linear palmar xanthomas are found in lipid abnormality Type III, obstructive jaundice and sometimes in Type IIa. Arcus senilis is due to lipid deposition in the cornea and, occurring under the age of 60, may be due to abnormal lipid metabolism. Hyperlipidaemia is investigated by measuring the fasting serum cholesterol and lipid levels and the estimation of lipoproteins by electrophoresis and ultracentrifugation. The WHO classification of lipid abnormalities, modified from Fredrickson, is used.

Classification of lipid abnormalities

Type I is the very rare Burger Gruz familial hyperchylomicronaemia, due to an absence of extrahepatic lipoprotein lipase. The chylomicrons in the blood produce milky serum, a very high level of serum triglycerides and lipaemia retinalis. The onset is in childhood as a rule. The liver and spleen are enlarged and there may be abdominal pain. There are eruptive xanthomata.

Type IIa hyperbetalipoproteinaemia (primary hypercholesterolaemia) is one of the commonest types of lipid abnormality. It is of autosomal dominant inheritance. The serum β-lipoproteins and usually the serum cholesterol are raised. Clinical manifestations are: tendon xanthomas, plane xanthomas, arcus senilis and ischaemic heart, peripheral vascular and cerebrovascular diseases.

Type IIb hyperlipoproteinaemia is also common. The pre-β-lipoproteins, the triglycerides and the cholesterol in the serum are raised. Xanthomata, cardiac ischaemia and obesity are clinical features.

Type III hyperlipoproteinaemia is rare. The serum cholesterol and triglycerides are usually raised and there is a broad

β-lipoprotein band on electrophoresis. There may be linear palmar and plantar xanthomas, tuberous xanthomas on the knees,
elbows and buttocks, tendon xanthomas and arcus senilis.
Ischaemic heart disease and peripheral vascular disease are also
clinical features.

Type IV hyperlipoproteinaemia is very common. The serum
pre-β-lipoprotein and triglyceride levels are increased. The cholesterol is normal or slightly raised. Xanthelasma is a feature.
Eruptive xanthomata occur rarely. Obesity, impaired glucose
tolerance and aggravation by alcohol may be features. A raised
incidence of cardiac ischaemia is disputed.

Type V hyperlipoproteinaemia is uncommon. There are raised
serum triglycerides with chylomicrons and sometimes a raised
cholesterol level. There is an increase in pre-β-lipoproteins shown
on electrophoresis. The clinical features include eruptive xanthomas, lipaemia retinalis, hepatosplenomegaly and attacks of
abdominal pain. Diabetes, alcoholism and the pill may be predisposing features.

Secondary xanthomatosis

Secondary xanthomatosis may result from diabetes, hypothyroidism, obstructive jaundice and alcoholism. The serum analyses
may not exactly fit the patterns of the lipid abnormalities Types
I–V.

The treatment varies between the different types: weight reduction
with a low saturated, high poly-unsaturated fat diet: drugs which
lower serum cholesterol, e.g. clofibrate; and, ion-exchange resins
which bind bile salts in the gut and prevent the resorption of
cholesterol, e.g. cholestyramine. The primary condition must be
treated in the secondary types of xanthomatosis.

Porphyria

The porphyrias form a group of disorders characterized by the
presence of abnormalities in the biosynthetic pathway leading to
the formation of haem. As a result various haem precursors called
porphyrins are formed in excess and spill out of the liver and bone
marrow. In excess, porphyrins are toxic to various organs, particularly the nervous system and skin. In the former they may cause
pain, peripheral neuritis, convulsions and coma. In the skin

porphyrins are photo-active, sensitizing the skin to 400 nm light and leading to skin damage. The porphyrias may be genetically determined or acquired. All are rare.

Erythropoietic protoporphyria

This condition begins usually in childhood and is the result of a dominant trait. Photosensitivity leads to blistering, scarring and thickening of the skin of the face and hands. Itching and 'burning' may be intense. Protoporphyrin levels are raised in the red cell series and plasma. The nervous system is not affected.

Porphyria cutanea tarda

In contrast this disease begins generally in the second half of life and is precipitated by liver damage, often due to alcohol. The exposed skin is liable to blistering, scarring and hyperpigmentation. It is excessively fragile and hypertrichosis develops on the face and brow. The affected skin may become sclerodermoid. Grossly abnormal amounts of uroporphyrins are excreted in the urine. The liver is demonstrably abnormal and there is excessive iron in it.

Treatment consists of withdrawing alcohol. Repeated venesection mobilizes excess iron from the liver and can induce clinical and biochemical remissions.

Variegate porphyria

This disease is inherited as a dominant trait and is very common in the white Africaner (Boer) population of South Africa. Both cutaneous and neuro-psychiatric manifestations are seen and the latter are particularly liable to be precipitated by certain drugs, particularly barbiturates and morphine.

Acute intermittent porphyria. This disease does not affect the skin.

GENETIC COUNSELLING

Parents are now able, more than ever before, to decide whether or not to have children and they will ask for medical advice about the risks of transmitting genetic disease. The first essential is an accurate diagnosis which, with an accurate family tree, should indicate the mode of inheritance. Autosomal dominant conditions carry a risk that 50% of offspring will be affected. The risk of transmission of autosomal recessive conditions is 25% but this risk is unlikely to be determined before the birth of an affected child. The risk of transmitting atopic eczema or psoriasis is less but cannot be predicted with the same accuracy. The risks can be explained sympathetically to the prospective parents who will themselves have to take the decision.

5

BACTERIAL DISEASES

The normal skin is inhabited by quite a large population of micro-organisms. Some of these are established and are called residents, e.g. diphtheroids and staphylococci. Others, especially on the exposed parts, are transients which do not multiply and do not persist. *Staphylococcus aureus* is carried on the skin by 20% or more of normal people; the nares, perineum and axillae are frequent carrier sites.

Impetigo

Impetigo begins in the subcorneal region of the epidermis and produces erythema and vesicles or bullae (Fig. 20). The vesicular type ruptures readily and produces stuck-on honey coloured crusts. These lesions may be circinate and resemble ringworm but the clinical course is more rapid. The bullous type ruptures less readily. The flaccid bullae are clear at first and later cloudy. Impetigo is usually asymmetrical and tends to affect the exposed parts, especially the face, the ears and the hands (Plate II). The organisms responsible are *Staphylococcus aureus*, the commonest cause in the United Kingdom, and the haemolytic streptococci. The latter is important in the United States and in the tropics and sub-tropics because it may cause nephritis. Impetigo is commoner in children than adults. It can occur in either healthy persons or it may be associated with pediculosis capitis, pediculosis corporis, scabies, eczema, or with poor hygiene, high humidity and small flies which can act as a vector, e.g. in Trinidad.

Treatment. If localized and accessible, impetigo should be treated with neomycin and gramicidin (Graneodin, U.K.), neomycin and bacitracin (Neobacrin, U.K.) or chlortetracycline ointment, four to six times a day. Widespread or inaccessible areas should be treated with oral antibiotics. Flucloxacillin or erythromycin are

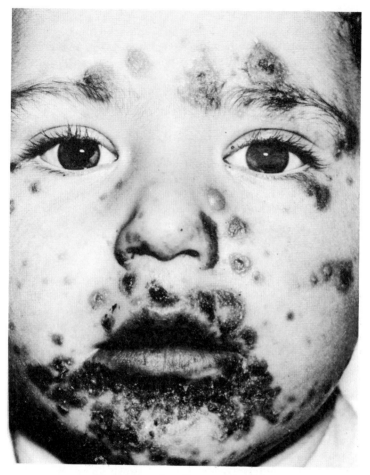

Fig. 20. Impetigo. (See also Plate II.)

advised when a penicillinase-producing staphylococcus is responsible. In parts of the world where streptococcal impetigo is common, routine oral treatment with penicillin may prevent nephritis.

Toxic epidermal necrolysis

Also called staphylococcal scalded skin syndrome or Ritter-Lyell disease, toxic epidermal necrolysis may be due to phage type 71 staphylococcal infection. It presents as an acute illness with redness and shedding of the outer layers of the skin. It is a serious disease and should be treated at once with flucloxacillin or erythromycin because the organism is resistant to ordinary penicillin and tetracyclines. Adverse drug reactions may produce a similar picture (see p. 148).

Erysipelas

Erysipelas is an acute, superficial, streptococcal infection which presents with bright red erythema, swelling and sometimes vesicles or bullae, which often have a distinct, palpable edge. Fever and rigors may also be evident. It is common on the face and on the legs (Plate III). There may be an obvious portal of entry of the organisms, e.g. a fissure at the angle of the mouth, in the entrance of the nose or ear, or between the toes.

Cellulitis

Cellulitis is a similar condition to erysipelas but deeper in the tissues, and therefore darker red and without vesicles. Penicillin or erythromycin by mouth is the treatment of choice. Portals of entry should receive appropriate treatment. Some people develop recurrent attacks of erysipelas or cellulitis at the same site leading to long lasting oedema. Long-term, daily administration of penicillin may be required.

Erysipeloid

Erysipeloid is an infection with *Erysipelothrix insidiosa* (formerly *Ery. rhusiopathiae*). It occurs in those who handle raw meat and fish and often follows a prick or scratch from a bone. A dull or purplish red, slowly spreading cellulitis, without constitutional symptoms, results. The erythema tends to spread down one finger and up another. The adjacent joints may also be affected. The treatment is penicillin V or oxytetracycline 500 mg four times a day for seven days.

Boils

Boils or furuncles are usually the result of the infection of a hair follicle with staphylococci. Boils of the head and neck are often associated with the nasal carriage of staphylococci and boils of the lower parts may be associated with axillary or perineal carriage. Other predisposing factors are scabies or other insect infestation, eczema, obesity and poor hygiene. Friction and maceration at the back of the neck and of the buttocks are also factors. The association with diabetes mellitus does not receive the same emphasis now as formerly. A boil may be a solitary abscess of the hair follicle, but more commonly they occur in crops, often in the same region, and they may become chronic. A multiple boil affecting adjacent hair follicles is a carbuncle. A boil of an eyelash follicle is a stye. Boils are a source of discomfort and ill health as well as being a source of contagion. They should be treated promptly and adequately with erythromycin or flucloxacillin for seven days, or for fourteen days or longer in chronic cases. The actual boils may be covered with adhesive plaster or may be treated with antibiotic cream or ointment (see Impetigo). An antiseptic soap should be used and chlorhexidine cream (Naseptin, U.K.) should be applied to carrier sites. Clothes should be changed and washed frequently. Underlying causes, such as scabies, eczema and obesity, should also receive attention.

Hidradenitis suppurativa

Hidradenitis suppurativa is an infection of the apocrine sweat glands of the axilla, groin or perineum. It is like a boil but even more unpleasant because the glands are deeper than most hair follicles. It should be treated with antibiotics as above but a longer course may be required. Anti-perspirants should be forbidden at the onset and for three months after recovery.

Sycosis barbae

Sycosis barbae is chronic folliculitis of the beard, usually due to *Staphylococcus aureus*. Since the advent of antibiotics it has become rare. In fact, nowadays most cases referred with this diagnosis have sterile folliculitis due to ingrowing hairs. There is also a fungal form of sycosis barbae (see p. 86).

Anthrax

Anthrax due to infections with *Bacillus anthracis* is primarily a disease of animals. It occurs in those handling imported, contaminated hides, wool and hair, e.g. tannery workers, dockers and also those who use bone meal as a fertilizer. The lesion usually begins on an exposed part, such as hands, arms, face or neck. A papule forms on the site of an abrasion and becomes surrounded with deep erythema. Bullae or vesicles form and become haemorrhagic. There is local oedema, lymphadenopathy and also fever. The diagnosis is confirmed by finding the large Gram-positive bacillus in the blister fluid and later by culture. Treatment with penicillin G, one million units four times a day by intramuscular injection or tetracycline intravenously at first, later by mouth 2 g per day for 14 days should be started promptly. Pulmonary and abdominal infections also occur.

Leprosy

Leprosy is due to infection with the acid-fast *Mycobacterium leprae*. It is no longer endemic in the United Kingdom but may be encountered in those areas where there is a high proportion of immigrants. The diagnosis should not be forgotten in those with non-itching skin disease or peripheral neuropathy who have spent time in countries where leprosy is endemic, viz countries bordering the Mediterranean, Africa, India, Burma, China, Malaysia, the Pacific Islands, central and southern America and the West Indies. Leprosy is usually acquired in childhood and the incubation period is often two to five years but may be longer. *Lepromatous leprosy* is the multi-bacillary 'open' type where a single blowing of the nose will produce 20×10^6 bacteria in a handkerchief. *Tuberculoid leprosy* is at the other extreme (Fig. 21). It is pauci-bacillary and often localized to one or two patches of skin and adjacent nerves. In between the two polar types is a spectrum of disease made up of the borderline and indeterminate varieties.

Lepromatous leprosy occurs in those with a poor immunological response. The lesions are macules, papules, nodules and plaques. Loss of sensation and neuropathy is a late finding. There may be localized alopecia of the beard and eyebrows. The nose and eyes may become involved. Tuberculoid leprosy presents as macules and plaques which are either red or hypopigmented. The lesions are often hypaesthetic to pin prick, touch and thermal sensation. Adjacent peripheral nerves are often enlarged and palpable.

A biopsy should be done and usually reveals characteristic histology. A skin smear should be made from the ear lobe or the edge of a lesion. An incision 2–3 mm deep and 5 mm long is made and the edges scraped with a scalpel. The material is put on a glass slide fixed with heat and stained with Ziehl-Neelsen stain. Numerous bacilli are found in lepromatous cases; it is rare to find bacilli in the tuberculoid. The lepromin reaction is not diagnostic; it is negative in lepromatous and positive in tuberculoid disease. Patients with open disease should be admitted to hospital but those with tuberculoid disease should be treated as outpatients.

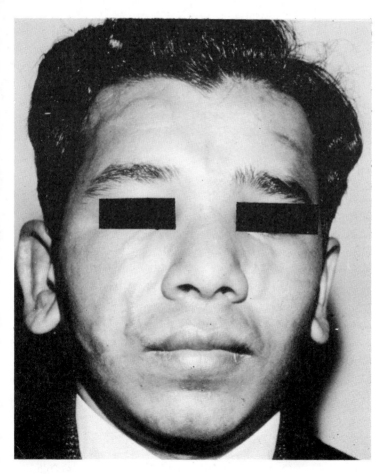

Fig. 21. Leprosy: tuberculoid or borderline type.

The main drugs used are dapsone (diaminodiphenyl sulphone), clofazimine and rifampicin. Although dapsone alone has been used with success for many years, the emergence of resistant strains of bacteria suggests that a combination of drugs should be used, at any rate in the lepromatous variety.

Leprosy is notifiable in the United Kingdom and the 'Panel of Leprosy Opinion' is available for advice. (Enquiries to the Leprosy Study Centre, 57A Wimpole Street, London W1M 7DF.)

TUBERCULOSIS OF THE SKIN

Tuberculosis of the skin, common at the beginning of the century, is now rare in advanced countries. The pasteurization of milk, the establishment of tuberculosis-free herds, improvements in housing and the development of effective treatment have brought about this happy state of affairs. However, it is still found in the United Kingdom, usually in immigrants of Asian origin.

Primary tuberculosis

Primary tuberculosis of the skin is less common than infection via the blood stream or lymphatics from within. The primary tuberculous chancre is an indolent ulcer with considerable regional lymph gland enlargement. *Lupus vulgaris* is the commonest type of infection (Fig. 22). It arises as a rule in patients who have an internal, pulmonary, glandular, abdominal or osseous infection. It usually begins in childhood or infancy and the head and neck (including the nose and inside the mouth) are common sites. The lesions are red-brown painless nodules which look like apple jelly when pressed with a glass spatula or slide. The nodules heal in the centre and scar, while fresh nodules are formed at the periphery. In extreme cases the nose may be destroyed and the palate perforated.

Warty tuberculosis

Warty tuberculosis (tuberculosis verrucosa cutis) is inoculation tuberculosis in people who are already partially immune from a previous infection. It is found on the hands and wrists of butchers, pathologists and postmortem workers and on the legs and buttocks of children. It looks like an ill-formed wart or keratotic plaque sitting on an area of cold erythema.

Bazin's disease

Bazin's disease (erythema induratum or tuberculous gumma) consists of indolent nodules on the legs of adolescent girls and young women. The nodules may ulcerate. A biopsy should be performed and a part sent for acid-fast bacillus culture and guinea pig inoculation. The chest should be X-rayed in all cases and a tuberculin test should be performed. Other systems presenting symptoms, such as the glands, bones and joints, should be investigated.

Although isoniazid alone has been shown to be an effective treatment, when the skin alone is infected it is usual to use com-

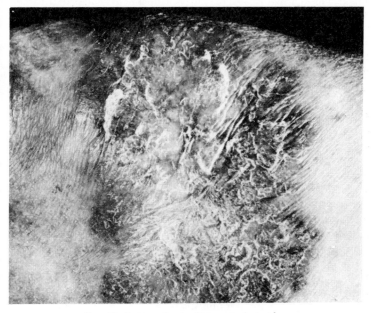

Fig. 22. Lupus vulgaris. Note central atrophy.

bined therapy, which prevents the development of drug resistance. The combined treatment is rifampicin, ethambutol and isoniazid for two months, followed by rifampicin isoniazid, sodium amino-salicylate isoniazid or ethambutol-isoniazid for nine months or for two months after clinical resolution.

Syphilis

Syphilis has now become relatively uncommon and, in consequence, doctors are no longer familiar with it and fail to recognize
the disease. Syphilis is still the original great imitator and should
constantly be borne in mind in diseases of the skin, mucosae, nails,
teeth, hair, not to mention the heart, the CNS and every other
system. The cause is an infection with the spiral organism *Treponema pallidum*, which enters the body through a break in the skin
or mucosa, travels to the regional lymphatic glands and later to all
parts of the body by the blood stream. The incubation period is
from nine to ninety days but usually twenty one to twenty eight
days. The disease is nearly always transmitted by sexual intercourse.

Primary syphilis

The portal of entry develops a primary chancre, a hard, indurated,
usually painless ulcer. The commonest site in men is the penis but
in homosexuals it may be the rectum, the anus or the perineum. In
women the vulva, the vagina and the cervix are the common
locations. Extragenital chancres may occur on the lip, inside the
mouth, on the tonsil, the nipple or on a finger tip. Those on the lip
or finger may be painful. The regional lymph nodes swell a few
days after the appearance of the chancre. The glands are discrete
and rubbery. The chancre heals spontaneously in a few weeks and
leaves a small scar. The differential diagnoses of the chancre
include simple inflammation of the glans penis (balanitis); herpes
simplex, which begins as close-set vesicles which rupture to form
erosions; chancroid, which presents with multiple painful ulcers
and is due to infection with *Haemophilus ducrei*; lymphogranuloma
venereum, which is a virus infection with tiny ulcers but very
significant regional lymph node enlargement and often suppuration; granuloma inguinale, a tropical venereal infection in which
Donovan bodies can be found histologically and which produces
a painless ulcer and later extensive granulation tissue; and,
carcinoma.

Secondary syphilis

Secondary syphilis usually follows within one to two months of the
chancre healing but it may begin earlier or later. The symptoms
may include headache, malaise, fever, lymphadenitis, anaemia,

skin and mucosal lesions and alopecia.. The rash is non-itchy, widespread, symmetrical and pleomorphic. The early macular and roseolar syphilide is pink and requires a warm room and a good light to detect it. The macules are round or oval and measure from 2 to 10 mm in size. The flanks and flexor surfaces of the arms are most affected. Coppery, raw ham or dusky red coloured papular rashes occur later. They are indurated and may become scaly, psoriasiform or pustular. The distribution is widespread and may include the palms and soles (Plate V). Condylomata lata are flat-topped moist raised masses, red or grey in colour. They are found in moist areas, around the anus, on the vulva or scrotum, around the mouth or between the toes. They swarm with treponemata. Papules in the mouth, the nose, the larynx, on the vulva, the cervix, the glans penis and in the anal canal are called mucous or moist patches. In the mouth these lesions may become eroded and form snail track ulcers. Patchy 'moth eaten' alopecia and widespread lymphadenopathy are also features. Macular and papular syphilides have to be differentiated from pityriasis rosea, seborrhoeic dermatitis, drug eruptions, rubella, scarlet fever, measles, psoriasis and lichen planus.

Tertiary syphilis

Tertiary syphilis, which is rare nowadays, may follow secondary syphilis in 2–10 years. The skin lesions are usually asymmetrical. Nodulo-ulcerative syphilides start as one or more nodules which break down and heal leaving tissue-paper scarring. Fresh lesions form a spreading semicircular front which may in time involve a considerable area. These lesions are very like lupus vulgaris but advance more rapidly. Some of the lesions are scaly and resemble psoriasis. Deep gummata may break through the skin and produce punched-out ulcers with a wash-leather base. The tongue may be affected, producing chronic superficial glossitis and leukoplakia.

Congenital syphilis

Congenital syphilis is transmitted across the placenta, hence there is no primary lesion. Early skin lesions may affect the palms, soles, the napkin area and around the mouth. The elements may be bullous, crusted or coppery and papular. Mucous patches and condylomata may be found. Scars radiating from the mouth (rhagades), frontal bossing of the skull and later Hutchinson's incisors and Moon's molars are also features.

Diagnosis and treatment of syphilis

Treponemata may be found in the exudate from the primary chancre and secondary lesions by dark ground microscopy. In the secondary and tertiary stages, the serological tests for syphilis are positive. The standard tests such as the Wassermann reaction and the Venereal Disease Research Laboratory Test (VDRL) are useful but they may give false positive reactions. If there is doubt, the *Treponema pallidum* haemagglutinin test (TPHA) should be used.

Procaine penicillin is given intra-muscularly in a dose of 1–2 g daily for 10–14 days. For those allergic to penicillin, oxytetracycline or erythromycin, 2 g per day for fifteen days by mouth, is recommended. The hazards of therapy include penicillin reactions and the Jarisch-Herxheimer reaction which is probably the result of the rapid destruction of a large number of organisms.

6

VIRAL DISEASES

Three of the common exanthemata of childhood are due to viruses, namely measles, varicella and rubella. They are not described in this chapter which is devoted to those viral infections where the skin is the main or sole organ involved.

HERPES ZOSTER

Herpes zoster, or shingles, is an acute, painful, self-limiting disease characterized by a unilateral and segmental eruption confined to one or more sensory dermatomes. It is due to the virus which causes chickenpox (varicella), and is a second clinical manifestation of infection which has remained latent in the tissues since an earlier chickenpox infection. Those who have had no visible lesions of chickenpox in childhood, and who yet develop zoster later in life have had a subclinical attack of varicella when young.

There are many well-authenticated cases of an adult having zoster and children in the same family developing varicella within the next three weeks. One attack of shingles usually confers immunity. Most persons who develop zoster are otherwise healthy, but there is a higher incidence in those with leukaemia and Hodgkin's disease.

The primary lesion of zoster is almost certainly in the sensory nerve supply of the affected part, but once the virus has entered the sensory neurone it passes peripherally to the skin and centrally to the neuraxis. The vesicles are due to direct action of the virus on the skin. The posterior root ganglion through which the sensory nerve supply passes is acutely inflamed, with round cell infiltration and haemorrhage. Degenerative changes occur along the posterior nerve root into the root fibres of the posterior columns of the cord, and along the course of the peripheral sensory nerves down to the fine fibrils in the skin at the site of eruption. Zoster affects the skin supplied by all the sensory fibres which pass through the diseased root ganglion. The vesicles are formed in the prickle-cell layer of the epidermis as a result of 'balloon degeneration' of the cells and serous exudation from the corium. The prickle cells of the affected areas swell in size, lose their attachments to other cells, and become separated. Their protoplasm becomes opaque, fibrinous and vacuolated. The nuclei increase in number and may contain oxyphilic inclusion-bodies. The balloon cells subsequently degenerate. There is some necrosis of the bases of the vesicles, and an invasion of leucocytes from the dilated blood vessels of the underlying corium.

Clinical picture

Zoster affects both sexes. It is seen mainly in the second half of life and is rare in children. Any dermatome may be affected but the thorax is the commonest site. In the aged, involvement of the first division of the trigeminal nerve is particularly common. Zoster of the maxillary division of this nerve is rare and of the mandibular division excessively rare. Disease of the thorax and lumbar segments is easily recognized, but cervical and sacral segment involvement may be missed because the rash is so localized.

Classically, the eruption is heralded by pain in a segmental distribution for up to a week. Patchy areas of erythema develop and quickly become oedematous. On these areas groups or clusters of papules erupt and rapidly become vesicular (Fig. 23). Crusts then form which separate in 14 to 28 days in the untreated disease. Secondary bacterial infection is unimportant. Enlargement of the draining lymph gland is usual. Sensory disturbance, including pain, paraesthesiae and numbness, persist in varying degrees throughout the attack and post-herpetic neuralgia may be a burden to which the aged are particularly liable. Zoster usually leaves scarring and pigmentation in its wake and, if the scalp is involved, cicatricial alopecia is not uncommon.

There are a number of clinical variants. Careful daily examination of the whole skin reveals sparse spattered varicella vesicles in 5% of patients, implying a viraemic phase. In immuno-suppressed patients and particularly in patients with Hodgkin's disease undergoing radiotherapy or chemotherapy, the typical eruption may evolve into confluent haemorrhagic and bullous zonal involvement. The affected area may become necrotic (gangrenous

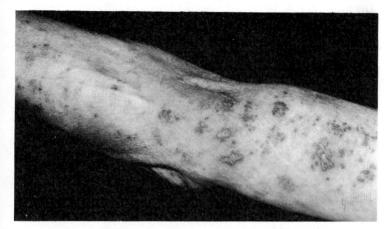

Fig. 23. Herpes zoster on arm. Note the grouping of the lesions.

zoster) and spread peripherally. A viraemia may lead to fatal varicella pneumonia or encephalitis.

As mentioned above, zoster involves the posterior horn of the spinal cord. Rarely, spread to the anterior horn results in motor involvement and paralysis. Complete paralysis of a limb is rare but usually permanent. Paralysis of other muscles may also occur, e.g. in the face or abdominal wall.

Mucous membranes may be involved, e.g. in geniculate zoster. In ophthalmic zoster (trigeminal, first division) involvement of the naso-ciliary branch implicates the conjunctivae.

Differential diagnosis

If the unilateral nature of zoster is borne in mind, diagnosis is rarely difficult. Ophthalmic zoster may cause oedema of both eyelids in the earliest stages, simulating contact dermatitis. Very localized zoster, e.g. on the genitalia, may mimic herpes simplex but, in the latter, pain of the same quality is unusual.

Treatment

If the disease is caught in the earliest stages, frequent application of 5% to 20% idoxuridine in dimethyl sulphoxide (DMSO) by painting the affected areas for three days will dramatically shorten the course of the disease and prevent much of the inflammation.

The lotion should be applied at least six times daily or even by continuous wet compress. It should not be used for more than three days, because DMSO is too irritant. It is contra-indicated in pregnancy. The higher the concentration of idoxuridine, the more effective the treatment is likely to be, but for large areas the cost is considerable. Once the inflammation is established, however, this treatment is useless and the application of 1% chlortetracycline in soft yellow paraffin is more valuable. Analgesic tablets may also be necessary. Topical steroids are contra-indicated but prednisolone, 40 mg daily by mouth, is highly effective if started early. The dose is reduced to zero over 10 – 14 days. This mode of treatment has never found favour in the United Kingdom but is widely employed in the United States and is of particular value in preventing post-herpetic neuralgia in the elderly.

HERPES SIMPLEX

This disease is one of the most ubiquitous viral infections of man. In the common recurrent form, localized herpetic eruptions occur which are unrelated to any dermatome but have the same morphology, though a shorter time course, than herpes zoster.

Aetiology and pathogenesis

Two types of herpes simplex virus have been identified: Type I and Type II. Type I is usually the cause of non-genital lesions, whereas Type II is usually transmitted venereally and affects the genitals. The two types are easily distinguished by their cultural and serological characteristics. Almost the entire adult population has been infected by Type I at some time although the infection is often sub-clinical. The vesicles of the clinical infection are found in the prickle-cell layer but no 'balloon' degeneration is seen. The viral inclusion bodies are oxyphilic and intra-nuclear.

The clinical picture: primary infections

Primary infections occur in individuals with no specific neutralizing antibodies; recurrent infections in those with such antibodies.

Primary herpes simplex infection is seen in infants from about 3 months of age, when the passive maternal antibodies wane, up to about 2 years. Most infections are sub-clinical. The clinical variants are:

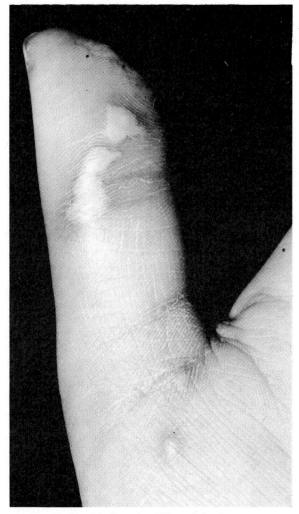

Fig. 24. Herpetic whitlow of thumb.

Primary herpetic gingivo-stomatitis. This infection is characterized by the sudden onset of painful oral lesions associated with fever, malaise and lymphadenopathy. The gingivae become red and swollen and erosions, blisters and superficial ulcers develop. The whole picture settles spontaneously in 7–14 days.

Primary herpetic vulvo-vaginitis is very similar to primary herpetic gingivo-stomatitis.

Inoculation primary herpes is due to direct implantation of the virus into the skin through an abrasion. It may be seen in wrestlers (herpes gladiatorum) and in doctors, dentists and nurses whose fingers encounter infected secretions, particularly from tracheostomy patients. The resulting so-called 'herpetic whitlow' is extremely painful and only slowly becomes vesicular (Fig. 24). Pus does not form.

Eczema herpeticum is one type of Kaposi's varicelliform eruption. It is a disseminated primary herpes occurring in a subject with atopic eczema (see p. 126). In small children it is alarming and may be fatal in a minority.

Neonatal infection is a hazard for the premature baby exposed to the virus in the birth canal. The viraemia induced is usually fatal.

The clinical picture: recurrent infections

Sufficient stress, e.g. prolonged high fever, will facilitate recurrent herpes simplex infection in many adults. Others suffer recurrent attacks, usually in one area, provoked by apparently trivial factors of which the most important are viral coryza (cold sore), minor fevers (fever sore), exposure to strong sunlight or local trauma. The eruption may be preceded for a few hours (or rarely a day or two) by tingling, burning or itching at the site. The erythema is followed by local oedema in which clusters of tiny vesicles, 1–3 mm in diameter, appear. Within three days, the vesicles become purulent and crusting follows. Involution takes 5 – 10 days and occasionally leaves slight scarring, especially after repeated attacks.

Recurrent herpes can occur anywhere but the common sites of Type I infection are the lips and peri-oral area (herpes labialis) (Fig. 25). Less commonly the chin or a cheek is involved. Extrafacial sites include the fingers, buttocks and thighs. Type I infections may occur within the mouth but are much more common in the eye as herpetic keratitis and dendritic corneal ulcer.

Recurrent Type II infections are common on the glans and shaft of the penis, although the site of recurrence often shifts slightly. Attacks are provoked by the trauma of coitus but usually settle in four or five days.

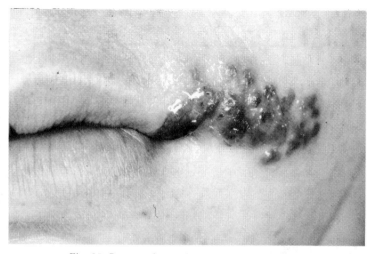

Fig. 25. Recurrent herpes simplex at corner of mouth.

Complications are unusual. Secondary bacterial infection is rarely a problem. Erythema multiforme may follow attacks by 10 – 20 days as an allergic response. In patients with severe immuno-suppression, induced by disease or drugs, the viraemia may be complicated by fatal pneumonia or meningo-encephalitis.

Treatment

In herpetic whitlow incision should be avoided. Continuous wet compressing with 5% to 20% idoxuridine in dimethyl sulphoxide (e.g. Herpid, U.K.) modifies and shortens the attack. In the rare, life-threatening herpes of infants, idoxuridine has been used intravenously but it is very toxic. Idoxuridine 0.5% eye drops are very useful in herpetic keratitis where steroids must be avoided, but the drug is less useful in recurrent skin infections. Herpid lotion is worth using if the patient presents on the first day of the eruption. It should be painted on the skin lesion four or five times daily for three days only. It does not prevent recurrence of lesions.

MOLLUSCUM CONTAGIOSUM

Molluscum contagiosum is a papular eruption of the skin caused by a pox virus which is transmitted either by direct contact or by fomites. Persons of all ages may be affected, but infection is commonest in children. Epidemics may occur in schools, orphanages or among patrons of Turkish baths. It may also be transmitted venereally. The virus causes proliferation of the prickle cell layer. The interpapillary processes of the epidermis grow downwards into the corium, compress the papillae into thin septa and form an epithelial mass. Under this mass the white connective tissue of the corium thickens to form a capsule and the small tumour rises above the surface of the surrounding skin. In the centre of the surface of the mollusc there is an opening which gives the tumour its typical umbilication. On microscopic examination, numerous large vacuolated cells with eccentric nuclei, containing closely packed eosinophilic hyaline bodies, are seen in the prickle cell layer.

Mollusca arise as minute painless elevations of the skin which slowly increase in size, usually reaching 2–3 mm in diameter. They may occur anywhere on the body but are usually seen on the upper trunk, neck and pelvic regions, sometimes in clusters. Their appearance is absolutely characteristic, as they form rounded, whitish elevations with an umbilicated centre, and frequently have a glistening, pearly white appearance (Plate VI). Pultaceous material may be expressed from them.

If left untreated the virus is conveyed on clothes, towels or fingers to other areas, so that groups of mollusca may be found all over the body. The lesions may be secondarily infected by scratching.

In rare cases spontaneous recovery occurs, but in the majority of cases the lesions, if untreated, are slowly progressive. The disease always yields to adequate treatment and causes no impairment of the general health.

The growths should be scraped out with a curette. Liquid nitrogen therapy may be effective. Alternatively, the lesions may be pierced with a spicule of wood which has been dipped in liquefied Phenol B.P. (80% phenol, w/w in water). Occasionally, general anaesthesia is needed to deal with a large number of lesions in a very young child.

WARTS

Warts, or verrucae, are cutaneous papillomata and may be regarded as localized, circumscribed hypertrophies of the prickle cell layer of the epidermis. The essential pathology of most

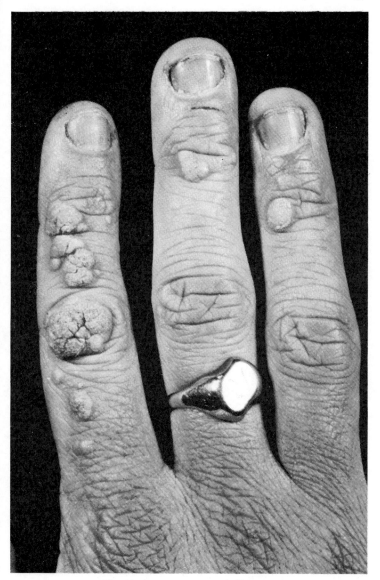

Fig. 26. Common warts on the fingers.

varieties is the same. Under the stimulus of a common agent, a papova DNA virus, the keratinocytes undergo active division resulting in a localized hypertrophy with acanthosis and hyperkeratosis.

There are six types of warts:

1. Common wart: *verruca vulgaris*.
2. Plane wart: *verruca plana*.
3. Digitate wart: *verruca digitata*.
4. Filiform wart: *verruca filiformis*.
5. Venereal wart: *condyloma acuminatum*.
6. Plantar wart: *verruca plantaris*.

Common warts are papilliferous excrescences which usually occur on the hands, but may occur elsewhere, especially on the face,

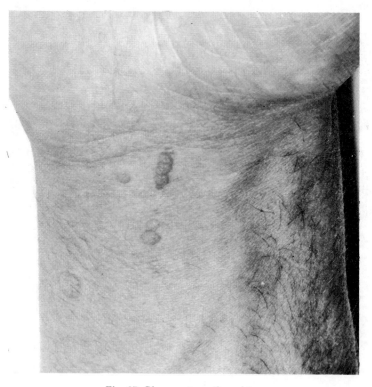

Fig. 27. Plane warts on the wrists.

knees and scalp. On the latter area the lesions frequently resemble cocks' combs. On the hands the lesions, which tend to enlarge peripherally, may extend round the nails. Unless cracked or infected they are symptomless (Fig. 26).

Plane warts are flat-topped, yellowish papules, 1–4 mm in diameter, formed by a localized acanthosis (Fig. 27). They occur chiefly on the backs of the hands, both aspects of the wrists and on the face and may itch. They occur mainly in young people and may persist for years. They may be sparse or present in scores, especially on the face. In men, they may disseminate widely in the beard area.

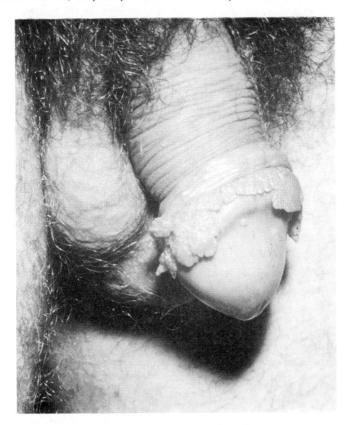

Fig. 28. Venereal warts on the penis.

Digitate warts are dark papillomatous excrescences, often topped by a black horny cap. Usually they grow on the head or neck.

Filiform warts are long and slender and grow on the eyelids, axillae or neck. They occur mainly in overweight, middle-aged women.

Venereal warts (condylomata acuminata) occur in the man on the penis (Fig. 28), often on the inner side of the prepuce and on the glans penis, especially at the balano-preputial groove. In women they are found on the vulva (Fig. 29) and may spread to the perineum. They are usually pink in colour, and may be small projections or exuberant cauliflower excrescences. They are often seen in patients suffering from other venereal diseases. Venereal warts rarely occur in childhood.

Plantar warts are most frequently seen in children and adolescents, but when present in adults can persist for years. They are readily contracted, and therefore minor epidemics readily occur in schools. The lesions are usually isolated and appear as little more than yellowish white, flattened, discrete, deeply imbedded, tender papules. If the surface of such a papule is pared away the papilliferous nature of the lesion is revealed. The lesion may be surprisingly deep as complete curettage reveals. Symptoms vary from the trivial to disabling tenderness on pressure and pain.

Occasionally an aggregation of these warts forms and spreads peripherally to make a dry, relatively painless, mosaic-like plaque, known as *mosaic warts* (Fig. 30).

TREATMENT

Common warts

Common warts are most easily treated by cryotherapy using liquid nitrogen (see p. 38). Small numbers of warts in the older child or adult may be curetted out and lightly cauterized under local anaesthesia. If surgery is undertaken for paronychial warts, care must be taken not to damage the nail matrix lest permanent nail deformity ensues. Only the lightest cauterization is advisable for warts at the tip of a digit since disabling painful scars may otherwise result. Destruction of common warts on the backs of the hands by electrical cauterization alone is not advised; it is much more painful than cryotherapy and leaves cosmetically unpleasant scarring. If, for any reason, the above modalities cannot be used or

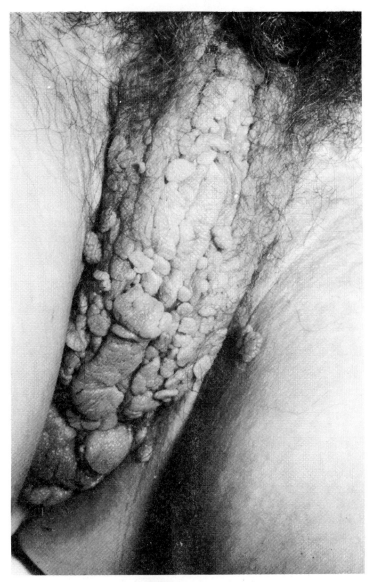

Fig. 29. Venereal warts on the vulva.

have failed, a lotion containing salicylic acid and lactic acid, 17% of each (Salactol and Duofilm, U.K. and U.S.A.), can be painted on the warts daily, allowed to dry and covered with an adhesive dressing. Other chemical approaches of less value include the daily application of 25% benzalkonium (Callusolve, U.K.) or 10% glutaraldehyde lotion (Glutarol, U.K.).

Plane, digitate and filiform warts

Plane warts are usually amenable to a series of light, weekly treatments with liquid nitrogen. Digitate and filiform warts should be snipped off and their bases lightly coagulated with electro-cautery.

Venereal warts

Venereal warts may be approached in several ways. Careful painting of the lesions with 15% to 25% podophyllin resin in tincture of benzoin, liquid paraffin or spirit is often rapidly effective. The podophylin must be applied by the doctor or nurse after the surrounding skin has been protected with soft paraffin and any excess mopped up. A gauze dressing is then applied to prevent spread and the application left on for 8 – 12 hours before being thoroughly washed off by the patient. If necessary, the treatment is repeated two or three times at weekly intervals. Podophyllin can be dangerous if used for very extensive vulval and introital warts in the pregnant woman because enhanced absorption of the resin may lead to severe neurotoxicity. More limited venereal warts can be treated by weekly application of 90% trichloracetic acid by the skilled operator and liquid nitrogen is useful for small spattered warts on the shaft of the penis. Occasionally excision, curettage and cautery under general anaesthesia are necessary for gross vegetating ano-genital warts. Lastly it should not be forgotten that other venereal infections, possibly transmitted at the same time, should be sought and sexual partners must be examined and treated if success is to be expected.

Plantar warts

Single, painful, tender plantar warts which are disabling the patient or preventing a child from school swimming are best curetted out under local anaesthesia. After the overlying hyper-keratosis has been pared away the wart is defined by blunt dissec-

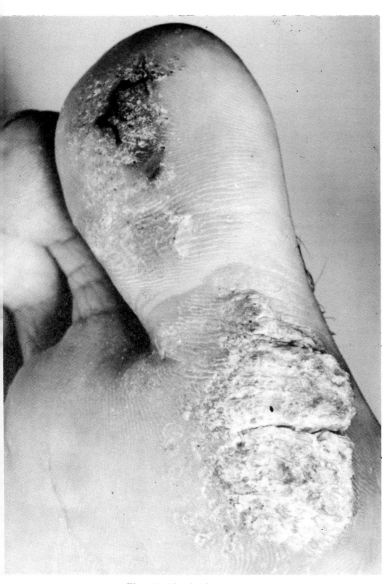

Fig. 30. Mosaic plantar warts.

tion and scooped out in one piece. After light electro-cautery of the sides of the wound a firm pressure dressing will control bleeding and need not be changed for five days. Relief of symptoms is usually instantaneous and healing uneventful in two to three weeks. The patient can walk normally from the second day. In skilled hands the cure rate is 80%.

In multiple plantar warts this approach is neither feasible nor worthwhile and daily soaking of the affected skin in 5% formaldehyde solution for 15 minutes daily is the treatment of choice. The solution is best prescribed as a 1 in 8 dilution of formalin, i.e. 5% formaldehyde in water. After 15 minutes, the foot is rinsed in plain water and dried. Dressings should not be applied. Only the affected skin should be exposed and the toe clefts may have to be protected with a smear of soft paraffin. The warts should be pared once a week using a corn plane. Three to four weeks of such treatment will produce cure in at least half the patients.

The various lotions mentioned above for common warts may have to be tried in plantar warts. Mosaic warts in the adult are particularly resistant to treatment and may persist for years. Adhesive plasters impregnated with 30% or 40% salicylic acid may be successful in their treatment; the plaster should be left on for 48 hour periods, alternating with 24 hour periods of rest. Sodden keratin must be regularly removed with a pumice stone or by sandpapering. Liquid nitrogen may also be useful for small or superficial plantar warts.

If plantar warts are symptomless or becoming less tender on lateral squeezing there is much to be said for doing nothing since more than 50% will disappear spontaneously in a few weeks. This is particularly so in very young children in whom the above procedures are difficult or impossible. In the authors' view it is only rarely justifiable to use general anaesthesia to deal with plantar warts surgically.

HAND, FOOT AND MOUTH DISEASE

This is a not uncommon infectious disease due usually to the enterovirus Coxsackie A16. Minor epidemics are common, the disease spreading rapidly amongst children and to adults within their families. After a four to six day incubation period an oropharyngeal exanthem appears. Transient vesicles give way to superficial ulcers, usually a few millimetres in diameter, which heal within a week. In two thirds of patients a characteristic exanthem follows the oral lesions by a day or so; rather sparse 3–7 mm superficial elongated vesiculopustules on an erythematous base are seen on the hands and feet and occasionally elsewhere. Like the mucosal lesions they heal within a week. These muco-cutaneous manifestations are accompanied in about 10% of patients by cervical lymphadenitis, coryza, diarrhoea, nausea or transient malaise. The virus can be cultured from the oral or cutaneous lesions to confirm the diagnosis directly or its presence can be inferred from rising serological titres in serial blood speci-mens. No treatment is available.

Differential diagnosis is from erythema multiforme. The foot and mouth disease of cattle is a separate disease due to a virus which rarely affects man. A number of other Coxsackie and Echo viruses can cause exanthems of various sorts.

PITYRIASIS ROSEA

This is a common disease of unknown aetiology characterized by a centripetal rash which lasts for several weeks. It is mainly seen between the ages of fifteen and forty years. It is probably slightly commoner in women. Second attacks are rare.

The first sign is a single erythematous oval or circular macule up to 3 or 4 cm in diameter. This is the 'herald patch' and it appears more often on the trunk than the limbs. The patch may become slightly scaly and may be 'ringed'. Itching is slight or absent. Within four to fourteen days, an exanthem follows in a centripetal distribution confined to the trunk, neck and the proximal parts of the limbs. The eruption is symmetrical and often particularly profuse about the shoulder girdle, including the axillae, and the pelvic girdle (see Fig. 15).

There are two components: the first, and the commoner, is characterized by lesions which have been described as 'medal-lions', and the second by small maculo-papules. Occasionally mixed varieties occur. A 'medallion' is an oval patch which, when fully developed, has a slightly raised peripheral zone, somewhat rose-coloured, with the colour of its outermost edge merging with the normal skin. The inner part of the peripheral zone shows fine scales which tend to be triangular in shape, the apices pointing inwards. The centre of the medallion is smooth, fawn-coloured and soft to the touch. Full evolution from a rosy macule to the complete lesion, which is often some 2 cm in its longest diameter, takes ten to fourteen days. The long diameters of the lesions on the back run downwards and outwards, producing an inverted Christmas tree pattern.

The lesions of the maculo-papular component are irregularly rounded, rose-pink, slightly elevated and covered after a few days with a fine scale.

The rash may take up to two weeks to fully develop. As it does so, the fine scaling becomes more marked, often forming a 'collarette' around the margin of individual lesions, with its edge facing the centre. The eruption then slowly fades away having run a total course of four to eight weeks.

Itching is variable and can be trivial or severe. Fierce attacks are rare but they may cause intolerable itching for a week or more. Malaise is rare. Giant, urticated and purpuric variants of pityriasis rosea are occasionally seen.

Differential diagnosis is important. The herald patch is often misdiagnosed as tinea. The fully developed eruption must be distinguished from seborrhoeic dermatitis, guttate psoriasis, drug eruptions and secondary syphilis.

The condition is almost uninfluenced by treatment and has to run its course. Oral antihistamines may allay itching and weak or medium corticosteroid creams may be of limited value.

OTHER VIRAL DISEASES

Orf

Orf is a virus disease of sheep and goats. In man it occurs only among those who handle these animals or their carcasses. The lesions are found most commonly on the fingers, hands and wrists. They begin as red papules, soon become vesicles, and eventually turn into pustules; sometimes the lesions are umbilicated. There are no constitutional symptoms, and the lesions disappear of their own accord in a few weeks.

Erythema infectiosum

This is a contagious disease of children also called fifth disease. It is probably due to an enterovirus. After an incubation period of 5–10 days, a characteristic exanthem appears on the face giving a 'slapped cheek' appearance. Later the erythema spreads widely, often in a lace-like pattern and lasts about two weeks. Constitutional disturbance is trivial.

Roseola infantum

This is a transient exanthem of toddlers, also called exanthema subitum and sixth disease. The responsible agent has not been identified. Fever, malaise and lymphadenopathy last two or three days and are followed by a very transient rubelliform rash. Neurological complications are not uncommon.

Gianotti-Crosti syndrome

This is a rare but distinctive syndrome, usually sporadic and seen in children. Over a few days a profuse papular eruption develops on the limbs and lasts a few weeks. There may be slight malaise, lymphadenopathy and splenomegaly. Minor abnormalities occur in the blood and liver function tests. The aetiology is unknown.

7

FUNGOUS DISEASES

The fungal infections of man are called mycoses. They can be simply classified as follows:–

Superficial mycoses	– ringworm (tinea)
	– candidiasis
	– tinea versicolor
Deep mycoses	– actinomycosis
	– sporotrichosis
	– blastomycosis, etc.

SUPERFICIAL MYCOSES

The superficial mycoses known as 'ringworm' are due to multicellular fungi, called dermatophytes, which form filaments or hyphae. Tinea versicolor and candidiasis are caused by unicellular fungi which reproduce by budding and are called yeasts.

Ringworm

The ringworm dermatophytes live in the stratum corneum of skin, hair and nail, i.e. the dead keratinized tissues which they can digest, but they cannot invade living tissue. Three genera are recognized called *Microsporon*, *Trichophyton* and *Epidermophyton*. Within these genera there are very many species of which about thirty are known to be pathogenic in humans. The dermatophytes can also be divided according to their sources. Anthropophilic species are restricted to man; zoophilic species are essentially pathogenic for animals but may infect man; geophilic species inhabit the soil and only rarely prove to be human pathogens.

Fungi vary in their ability to invade skin, hair or nail and in their capacity to excite an inflammatory reaction in the host. Zoophilic species tend to cause much more inflammation than anthropophilic ones.

In the host tissue, the filamentous hyphae of dermatophytes segment into chains of arthrospores which are responsible for spread of infection. On suitable tissue, these spores germinate into more hyphae, spreading along the outer epidermis and invading any hair follicles that are present. Some species have the ability to penetrate the hair shaft within the follicle and spread down against the direction of hair growth until the living tissue of the hair bulb arrests further penetration. In an anagen follicle, the fungus may invade newly formed hair indefinitely, perpetuating the infection until the follicle goes into the telogen, or resting, phase. Subsequent shedding of the telogen hair spontaneously 'cures' the infection in that follicle.

Growth of the hair in an infected follicle passively carries the fungus back to the skin surface and beyond. If the infected shaft is weakened, it may break, providing a source of potentially infectious material. In some species the arthrospores are formed outside the hair shaft in the infected follicle; this is called ectothrix infection. In others, the arthrospores only form inside the hair shaft, and these are called endothrix spores. The importance of the distinction between endothrix and ectothrix infections for the clinician is that ectothrix spores are associated with the deposition

TABLE 1. Main Species of Pathogenic Fungi

Genus	Species	Source	Main Site	Wood's Light
Microsporon	M. audouini	human	scalp	positive
	M. canis	animal	scalp	positive
Trichophyton	T. rubrum	human	nails, hands, feet, groin	negative
	T. interdigitale	human	feet, groin	negative
	T. mentagrophytes	animal	body	negative
	T. sulphureum	human	scalp	negative
	T. violaceum	human	scalp	negative
	T. schoenleinii	human	scalp	positive
	T. verrucosum	animal	body	negative
Epidermophyton	E. floccosum	human	feet, groin	negative

of a fluorescent chemical on the outside of the hair shaft which can be detected by Wood's light examination. Thus, ectothrix infections are Wood's light positive, endothrix infections are not.

The most important species in the U.K. are summarized in Table 1. *Trichophyton rubrum* is now predominant, with *Trichophyton mentagrophytes* var. *interdigitale* and *Epidermophyton floccosum* in second and third place. Infection is much commoner in males at all sites except the lower leg and ankle.

It is convenient to describe the clinical patterns of tinea by site.

TINEA CAPITIS (RINGWORM OF THE SCALP)

Tinea capitis may be caused by *Microsporon* or *Trichophyton* fungi. *Microsporon* infections are seen mainly in childhood and are of two types: *Microsporon audouini*, which spreads from child to child and may cause epidemics in schools and other institutions; and *Microsporon canis*, which is acquired from kittens and puppies and occurs sporadically. *Trichophyton* infections occur in adults and may be of several types, presenting a variety of clinical pictures.

The common *Microsporon* tinea of the child's scalp commences in one or more areas of the scalp as a small, ovoid, scaly patch which spreads at the periphery and may involve the whole of the hair-bearing area (Fig. 31). On examination the affected part is seen to be covered with broken-off, lustreless hair stumps 1–2 mm in length. There may also be scaling of the skin. Hair stumps and scales should be collected with a scalpel or epilating forceps, wrapped in paper and sent to the mycologist for microscopical examination and culture. Viewed under Wood's light in a dark room the affected hairs on the scalp fluoresce a brilliant green.

Scalp ringworm due to *Trichophyton* fungi often presents a different clinical picture. In one type the hairs are broken off at the point of their emergence from the scalp, which gives the appearance of small black-heads on the scalp and the name 'black-dot ringworm'. In another type, usually contracted from animals, the patient exhibits raised boggy swellings on the scalp, where the follicles ooze sero-pus. The suppuration in the follicles causes the hair to fall out, and the disease is self-curative. Small local areas of permanent baldness with depressed scars, sometimes pitted with sunken follicular orifices, may be left. This is called kerion and the suppuration is the consequence of the body's reaction to the fungus

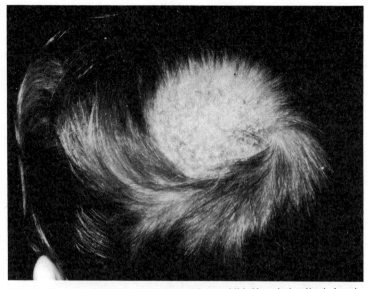

Fig. 31. Tinea capitis (Microsporon canis) *in a child. Note the localized alopecia and scaling.*

and is not due to secondary infection. If abscesses on the scalp are bacteriologically sterile the pus should always be cultured for fungi. Most *Trichophyton* infections of the scalp do not fluoresce under Wood's light; non-fluorescence does not exclude tinea.

Favus is a distinct form of tinea capitis due to *Trichophyton schoenleinii* in which affected hairs do fluoresce a dull grey-green colour. It is rare in north west Europe. Untreated, favus pursues a chronic course eventually leading to extensive cicatricial alopecia. In the early stages characteristic concave crusts, or scutula, are seen. Infected hairs do not break easily and long lengths may fluoresce.

Differential diagnosis is from alopecia areata and traumatic alopecia due to traction or friction.

If culture reveals *M. audouini*, the source of infection should be sought within the family, friends or school, if necessary enlisting the help of the school medical officer. Large numbers of children can be screened quickly by Wood's light examination. The patient must be kept away from school until cured. In *M. canis* infections the animal source should be identified and treated.

The diagnosis of non-fluorescent *Trichophyton* infections can be confirmed by microscopy and culture of scalp scrapings or 'hair brush' specimens. Griseofulvin is the treatment. In acute kerion, use of the antibiotic is supplemented by daily removal of loose hairs with forceps.

Treatment. Microsporon tinea of childhood cannot be treated by topical fungicides., Before the antibiotic griseofulvin became available in 1959, X-ray epilation was the routine treatment. Griseofulvin is given by mouth once daily after the main meal. The dose is one 500 mg tablet for adults and 250 mg or 375 mg, as 125 mg tablets or a suspension, for children. Treatment must be continued for at least two months and until Wood's light examination is negative. A fungicide cream can be applied twice daily.

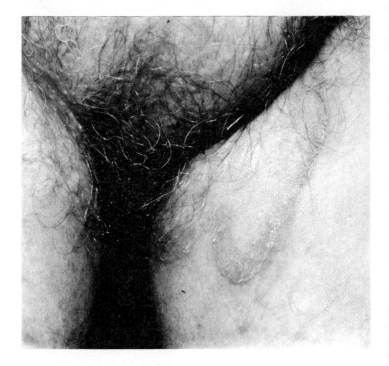

Fig. 32. Tinea cruris.

Tinea Corporis (Ringworm of the Glabrous Skin)

The often ringed lesions of tinea corporis give the disease its name. The eruption is typically sparse and asymmetrical with one or more erythematous, scaly, discoid lesions, each sharply defined and spreading slowly centrifugally. In some types there may be marginal vesicles or pustules. Itching is variable. The infection is often of animal origin.

Treatment. Topical fungicides will often suffice for mild infections. For more serious infections a three week course of griseofulvin is curative.

Tinea Cruris (Ringworm of the Groins)

The intertriginous inguinal fold is a favourite site of tinea caused by *E. floccosum*, *T. mentagrophytes* var. *interdigitale* or *T. rubrum*. The first two are virtually only seen in the male but tinea cruris due to *T. rubrum* also occurs in the female, albeit uncommonly. *E. floccosum* infections only spread locally on the upper inner thighs to produce a sharply defined 'butterfly' rash more inflamed at its margins (Fig. 32). The margin of the rash may be vesicular, pustular or scaly. *T. rubrum* infections often spread much more widely if not treated, extending to the mid thighs, through the perineum and onto the buttocks (Fig. 33), posterior thighs or the lower abdominal wall. The margin is scaly but never vesicular.

The natural appearance of tinea cruris is often masked by inappropriate topical steroid therapy which partially suppresses the inflammation and encourages its spread. The distinct margin of the infection is broken up and deeper, inflammatory, 'boil-like' lesions may be seen. The name 'tinea incognito' has been applied to this iatrogenic variant.

Differential diagnosis is from simple eczematous intertrigo, flexural psoriasis and seborrhoeic dermatitis, all of which are more symmetrically distributed above and below the inguinal creases. Candidiasis is much commoner in the female and is characteristically vesicular or papulo-pustular with outlying 'satellite' lesions. Erythrasma (p. 95) is a more macular low grade inflammation which fluoresces coral-pink under Wood's light. The diagnosis of tinea cruris is confirmed instantly by direct microscopy of unstained scrapings. The causative dermatophyte is identified by culture.

Treatment. The inflamed groin does not tolerate 'strong' local applications and it is easy to induce a secondary contact dermatitis by injudicious topical therapy. Strong topical steroids, if being used, must be withdrawn. If the area is acutely inflamed, 1:8000 potassium permanganate compresses for 10 minutes twice daily for two days and then daily for three days are invaluable. After this compress, the skin is gently dabbed dry and a cream containing an iodoquinoline antiseptic and a weak corticosteroid (e.g.

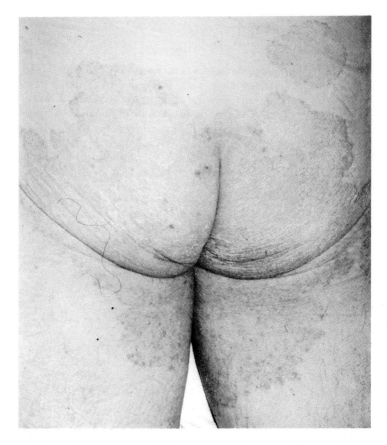

Fig. 33. Tinea cruris due to Trichophyton rubrum *spreading posteriorly.*

Vioform-Hydrocortisone, U.K.) applied twice or thrice daily. Later, as the inflammation subsides, clotrimazole or miconazole nitrate creams can be substituted. In severe infections and in all *T. rubrum* infections a three to four week course of griseofulvin is indicated. In the latter situation a non-irritant, topical fungicide can be used from the beginning of treatment.

TINEA PEDIS (RINGWORM OF THE FEET)

Tinea pedis (Fig. 34) is common and caused by the same three species which cause tinea cruris. It is much more common in males than females and is uncommon in young children. The infection is transmitted via swimming bath, shower, changing room and bathroom floors. Shoes and socks are important sources of re-infection.

There are three main clinical patterns:

1. Intertrigo occurs especially between the fourth and fifth toes. The toe cleft skin is sodden and white and rubs off to leave raw red areas.

2. Vesicular patterns usually due to *T. interdigitale* begin on the sides of toes or on the instep, side or dorsum of the foot. Vesicles, bullae or pustules may be seen. The lesions rupture, dry and leave collarettes of scale. Very acute vesicular tinea is occasionally complicated by secondary allergic vesicular eczema, or pompholyx, on the remainder of the soles and the palms; the so-called 'id' reaction.

3. In the hyperkeratotic pattern, diffuse or patchy thickening of the sole is seen. The surface may or may not be reddened but is usually finely exfoliative and the skin creases are accentuated by white scale. This is a chronic pattern almost always due to *T. rubrum*. It is commonly associated with an infection of the toe nails.

Differential diagnosis is from endogenous eczema, contact eczema due to footwear and psoriasis. Toe cleft intertrigo is sometimes due to candidiasis, erythrasma or simple maceration.

Treatment. The mild intertriginous type responds to twice daily application of any efficient topical fungicide, e.g. Whitfield's ointment. Attention should be paid to foot hygiene and the avoidance of excessively occlusive toe environments. Severe intertrigo responds to 1:8000 potassium permanganate compresses and Vioform-Hydrocortisone cream (U.K.) as for acute tinea cruris, followed by resort to other topical fungicides. The same manage-

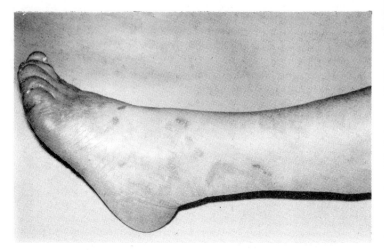

Fig. 34. Extensive tinea pedis spreading to ankle and calf.

ment is appropriate for severe or acute vesicular patterns, although these may be complicated by coccal infection requiring an oral antibiotic. Hyperkeratotic *T. rubrum* infections need a three month course of griseofulvin, together with nightly application of Whitfield's ointment or miconazole nitrate cream (Dermonistat, U.K.).

Tinea Barbae (Ringworm of the Beard)

Tinea barbae is mostly seen in rural areas and is acquired from farm animals. *Trichophyton verrucosum* and *T. mentagrophytes* are commonly responsible. Occasionally tinea barbae may be contracted from a cat or dog, when the fungus is *Microsporon canis*. Human to human spread, commonly with *T. rubrum*, also occurs. In the past the condition was called 'barber's itch' because it was disseminated by barbers' shops.

The disease commonly attacks localized areas, though it may, of course, spread over the whole of the beard area, although the upper lip is seldom affected. In the severe form acquired from farm animals the hair follicles are invaded, and a suppurative condition is set up. The affected area appears as a mass of small boils, at the apex of which a broken-off hair projects through a bead of pus, which comes from the hair follicle. In less severe cases 'lumpy' swellings may be found, and no pus is visible. In the least severe cases where infection is acquired from man, cat or dog, a few broken-off hairs are found.

Differential diagnosis is from staphylococcal folliculitis and depends on microscopy of hair and scales, and fungal and bacteriological cultures.

Treatment. Griseofulvin for three weeks is indicated. With kerion, loose hairs should be epilated daily. A fungicide cream can also be used.

TINEA MANUUM (RINGWORM OF THE HAND)

T. rubrum is usually responsible for ringworm of the hand. Five clinical patterns are recognized:

1. Vesicular discoid patches.
2. Crescentric exfoliating scaling lesions as seen on the soles (Fig. 35).
3. Discrete red papular and follicular scaly patches on the backs of the hands or wrists.
4. Erythematous scaly sheets on the backs of the hands.
5. Hyperkeratotic erythematous finely exfoliative sheets as on the soles. This pattern is confined to the palmar aspect of the hand and is often unilateral.

Differential diagnosis is from endogenous and contact eczema and psoriasis.

Treatment. Griseofulvin is usually indicated. Three to four weeks suffice for infections of the back of the hand but eight weeks treatment should be given for hyperkeratotic parmar infections. In addition Whitfield's ointment or miconazole cream can be used.

FOLLICULAR TINEA OF THE CALVES

Often clinicians fail to recognize that certain unusual eruptions on the lower two-thirds of the legs may be due to infection with *T. rubrum*. These are not necessarily accompanied by tineal infection of the toe-webs and toes. The infection is usually seen in women.

Usually the lesions are irregularly shaped, unilateral, mildly erythematous patches covered with small maculo-papules or showing a folliculitis. Occasionally erythema nodosum-like nodules are seen.

Treatment is by means of griseofulvin and anti-fungal ointments.

Tinea Unguium

Fungal infection, usually with *T. rubrum*, is commoner in the toe nails than the finger nails. It is also called ringworm of the nails or onychomycosis. The infection begins at the free end of the nail, often laterally, and gradually extends proximally until the whole

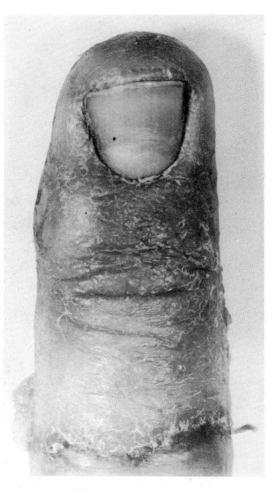

Fig. 35. Tinea of the finger.

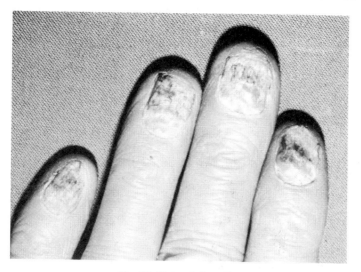

Fig. 36. Tinea of the nails.

nail plate is diseased. The affected nail loses its lustre and becomes brittle and opaque. Its surface becomes roughened and eventually the nail may become grossly thickened or crumble (Fig. 36). Paronychia is not a feature.

Differential diagnosis is from psoriasis and candidiasis.

Treatment. In general, toe nail infections in the adult due to *T. rubrum* are incurable. Prolonged courses of griseofulvin lasting four to eight months can cure finger nail infections but, clearly, such therapy should not be undertaken unless the diagnosis has been confirmed by microscopy and culture.

Candidiasis (Moniliasis)

Candidiasis is an infection of skin, nails and mucosae usually caused by the yeast, *Candida albicans*, although rarely other *Candida* species are implicated. The yeast is a normal resident of the gastrointestinal and genital mucosae which only becomes pathogenic when an opportunity arises. A number of clinical situations provide such an opportunity, for example pregnancy, oral contraceptive therapy, wide-spectrum antibiotic therapy, oral or topical corticosteroid therapy, immunosuppressive drug therapy, endocrine disorders such as diabetes mellitus and hypoparathyroidism and blood dyscrasias. The disease is seen at the extremes of life, i.e. in the neonate's mouth as thrush, before the normal antagonistic bacterial flora have become established, and in the very old or debilitated. It may also be seen in patients suffering from malnutrition. In extreme situations systemic infection is possible with candidial endocarditis, meningitis or lung infections which may be fatal.

There are several clinical patterns of candidiasis which can be seen.

Thrush

Thrush is oral candidiasis which presents as whitish patches on the buccal mucosa. These patches are easily scraped off to reveal an inflamed mucosal surface. The tongue and lips may also be involved.

Angular stomatitis

Angular stomatitis involves the skin and mucosae of the corners of the mouth and may be complicated by painful fissuring. It may be the result of sagging of the face in older people with dentures, leading to the formation of an intertriginous fold.

Balano-posthitis

Balano-posthitis due to *Candida* is a common presenting feature of diabetes in men. Alternatively it may be caused by candidial vulvo-vaginitis in the sexual partner.

Vulvo-vaginitis

Vulvo-vaginitis is common in pregnancy and diabetes and is a recognized complication of oral contraceptive therapy. It may occur when girls on 'the pill' are being given long-term oral tetracycline for acne vulgaris. The infection causes vulval pruritus with variable rash and characteristic vaginal discharge. In severe infections the vaginal walls show the features of oral thrush.

Intertrigo

Intertrigo in the sub-mammary, abdominal, ano-genital or inter-digital folds between the third and fourth finger (erosio interdigitalis) is often partially or even wholly due to *C. albicans* in the presence of predisposing factors. The eruption is moist and erythematous with a well defined margin which is often scaly or pustular. Outlying, 'satellite' papulopustules may be seen. Occasionally pruritus ani is caused in the absence of obvious intertrigo.

Chronic paronychia

Chronic paronychia is a low grade infection of the finger nail folds, which become tender, painful, swollen and red (Fig. 37). A cheesy discharge may be expressed from the open space between the cuticle and the nail plate. *Candida* is usually the main organism involved but bacterial infection may also be present.

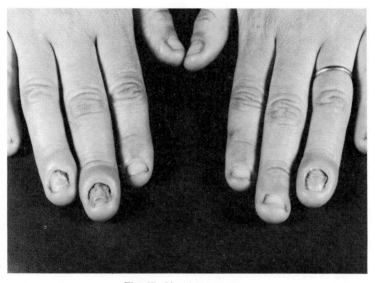

Fig. 37. Chronic paronychia.

The infection is most common in women, particularly those with a rather poor peripheral circulation. In this situation, the vitality of the cuticles can be undermined by repeated exposure to detergents, soaps, solutions of soda, cuticle removers and cosmetics. The right hand is most frequently affected. When the cuticle barrier is broken, the cuticles cease to be formed and infection of the para-ungual tissues readily occurs.

Sometimes the infection is active and the inflammatory changes acute, whilst at other times the inflammation passes into a sub-acute or chronic state. If it persists for a long time, as it usually does, transverse ridging of the infected nails may be seen. Candidial infection of the nails may also be present, indicated by loss of translucency, fragility and often a characteristic greenish-brown discoloration of the nail plates. In differential diagnosis, the possibility of streptococcal or staphylococcal infections of the paronychial tissues should be remembered. However, in both these cases the inflammation is acute, may be associated with cellulitis or lymphangitis and is a relatively virulent infection.

Onychia

Candidial infection of the nail plate is particularly seen in hypoparathyroidism and in certain rare states of immune deficiency. The nail plate may be grossly disorganized.

Differential diagnosis of candidial intertrigo is from tinea, seborrhoeic dermatitis, flexural psoriasis, pyoderma and contact dermatitis. The diagnosis is confirmed by microscopy of skin or mucosal scrapings which reveals small oval budding yeasts which may grow into filaments. Culture is less valuable since it may pick up harmless commensals.

Treatment

Underlying predisposing factors should be dealt with as far as possible. A number of preparations are available which are very active against *C. albicans*, e.g. the antibiotics nystatin and amphotericin B, the iodoquinolines (chinoform, clioquinol, chlorquinaldol), clotrimazole (Canesten, U.K.) and miconazole nitrate (Daktarin, Dermonistat, U.K.). Gentian violet, 0.5% or 1% in water, is also effective.

Nystatin and amphotericin are available as lozenges for the treatment of oral lesions and as pessaries for vaginal treatment. All are available as creams or ointments for treatment of the skin. Nystatin tablets, one twice daily, are effective in the gastro-intestinal tract and occasionally are useful for candidial pruritus ani or where recurrent genital infection in the female is thought to originate from the lower bowel. Nystatin is not absorbed from the gut and in the rare systemic infections, amphotericin B must be given intravenously. Griseofulvin is inactive against *Candida*.

Tinea Versicolor

Tinea versicolor or pityriasis versicolor is caused by *Malassezia furfur*. The mycelium of *M. furfur* attacks only the stratum corneum and on microscopical examination is seen to consist of short rod-like or bent pieces of fine mycelium, between which lie grape-like clusters of round or oval spores.

The malady is slightly contagious but is seldom seen in children. It is particularly common in the tropics or sub-tropics and may be acquired on a holiday there. Systemic and topical steroid therapies predispose to this infection, as in candidiasis.

On the skin of Caucasian races the first sign is the appearance of irregular, fawn or brownish, slightly scaling macules which coalesce to form irregular figures. Large areas of skin may be involved but the neck, shoulders, upper trunk and upper arms are the usual sites (Fig. 38). The patches have well-defined borders, but healthy skin lies between them. Often the appearance is like a map with continents and islands painted on the skin in light-brown pigment. In coloured persons, and sunburned Caucasians, depigmentation of the infected skin may occur (achromia parasitica) and the infected areas look like the patches of leucoderma seen in vitiligo. Examination of the patient under Wood's light shows faint orange, gold or buff fluorescence in the affected areas.

It may be difficult to differentiate between tinea versicolor and vitiligo but close examination almost always reveals slight inflammation and fine scaling, which are absent in vitiligo. Usually, it is easy to demonstrate the mycelium and spores in scrapings taken from the lesions of this type of fungous infection. They should be mounted as wet specimens in 5% potassium hydroxide solution and examined microscopically under the one-third or one-sixth objective.

Treatment

Six daily applications of 2.5% selenium sulphide suspension (Selsun, U.K.) are usually curative. The suspension should be applied to the whole trunk, neck and arms and washed off after one hour. Alternatively, clotrimazole (Canesten, U.K.) or miconazole

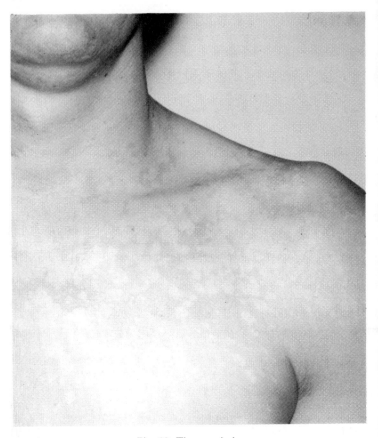

Fig. 38. Tinea versicolor.

nitrate creams (Daktarin or Dermonistat, U.K.) can be applied twice daily for 10 days. Griseofulvin is of no value in the treatment of tinea versicolor.

There may be a reservoir of infection in the scalp which is best dealt with by three or four applications of Selsun, U.K., for 15 minutes each time the hair is washed. Clothing worn next to the affected skin should be washed or dry cleaned before being re-worn after treatment. When pigmentation is disturbed the patient must be told that this will take much longer to settle.

Erythrasma

In Britain, erythrasma is seen as a form of intertrigo, characterized by slightly scaling, dry, irregularly shaped areas, reddish brown in colour, which extend peripherally and may become concurrent. The infection is usually seen in the groins or axillae, but sometimes affects folds of abdominal skin or the submammary areas.

The lesions fluoresce coral-red or brown-violet under Wood's rays, and examination by this means has suggested that the incidence of this infection in the 'normal' population is higher than is usually thought.

The cause has now been proved to be infection by *Corynebacterium minutissimum*, which produces a porphyrin that is responsible for the fluorescence under Wood's light. *Corynebacterium minutissimum* is usually sensitive to erythromycin and the tetracyclines. Erythromycin is said to be the antibiotic of choice, and should be given in doses of 250 mg four times daily for five days; this quickly clears erythrasma from all areas except the toe-webs, where Whitfield's ointment should be used.

The Deep Mycoses

Actinomycosis

Actinomycosis is an infective granuloma characterized by the formation of nodules, which ulcerate and discharge a typical pus. The disease occurs on the skin, but may commence in other tissues; it may spread by metastasis to any part of the body. It is caused by *Actinomyces*, of which *Actinomyces israelii* is the cause of about 90% of the cases in man. *Actinomyces* are anaerobic fungi which often live saprophytically in the mouth and gastrointestinal tract of animals and man; under certain conditions the organisms become pathogenic. The incubation period is unknown, but possibly varies from a few days to several weeks. Adults are more frequently affected than children, and men than women.

Signs and Symptoms. The face, neck, chest and abdomen are the most commonly affected, though the lesions, which are relatively painless, may erupt on any part of the body. In Britain, a solitary abscess on the cheek of dental origin is one of the commoner presentations. Infection may occur through an abrasion in the skin, but happens much more often through the mucous membrane of the mouth, from which the disease spreads to the skin. Lesions on the knuckles caused by punching someone in the mouth have been described. When the abdominal skin is involved the infection is often a sequel to an operation on the caecum or appendix.

The disease commences by the appearance of a subcutaneous nodule which enlarges, suppurates, forms an abscess, and then bursts, discharging a pus which contains greenish-grey or sulphur-coloured granules. These granules consist of small colonies of the *Actinomyces*. In rare instances, as one nodule enlarges another forms in close apposition to it, and the clinical picture thus obtained is of a mass of nodules surrounding an ulcerated area. The nodules are frequently as large as a hazel-nut, and on palpation of the affected area one is impressed by the board-like resistance which one's finger encounters. The disease spreads inwards and may involve the bone, in which case a very intractable sinus results and the prognosis becomes less optimistic.

The disease must be differentiated from the other infective granulomata. The clinical diagnosis should be confirmed by microscopical and cultural examination of the pus, which has to be carefully searched for the granules. Precipitating antibodies can be sought by serological methods.

Treatment. Penicillin, one of the tetracyclines or erythromycin may be used. The doses must be high, and treatment usually prolonged, for example, 0.5 to 1.0 mega units of penicillin thrice daily for six weeks or more, or one of the tetracyclines 750 mg four times daily for 14 days and then standard dosage for several weeks. Cephalothin and clindamycin have been used successfully in recent reports.

Chromoblastomycosis

This is a chronic, slowly progressive fungal infection of the tropics, only rarely seen in northern Europe. It is caused by *Phialophora* and *Cladosporium* species and may spread metastatically. It is characterized clinically by the development of warty nodules on the skin, usually on the legs or buttocks. Large plaques and tumours may form. Differential diagnosis is from other infective granulomata. The diagnosis is confirmed by histological and cultural examination of biopsy material.

Treatment is unsatisfactory. Localized lesions may be excised. Therapeutic claims have been made for isoniazid, thiabendazole and 5-fluorocytosine used systemically. Amphotericin B can be used intra-lesionally. The disease can recur after long periods of quiescence so the prognosis must be guarded.

Sporotrichosis

Sporotrichosis is a contagious disease caused by a fungus and characterized by the formation of nodules which may occur, not only in the skin, but in almost any organ or tissue in the body. The nodules break down and, on the skin, form comparatively painless ulcers. The disease is more common on the Continent than in England.

Sporotrichosis is caused by *Sporotrichum schenckii*, which may be contracted from plants and vegetables, as well as from man and birds. The fungus is easily cultivated in Sabouraud's medium.

Signs and Symptoms. The patient complains of 'ulceration of the skin'. On examination small nodules are found, which appear to lie in the subcutaneous tissues. These enlarge, become red and form small abscesses which burst causing indolent ulcers, irregular in outline, with undermined and inflamed edges. The disease tends to spread by the lymphatics, and a significant feature is the development of a series of ulcers extending from a primary sore, which often develops at the site of a minor injury, up a limb in the line of the lymphatic drainage. Rarely sporotrichosis disseminates via the blood stream and not by the lymphatics; this is usually fatal.

Occasionally only one chronic sore, with no metastases, develops. It is usually on an area exposed to injury, and may take various forms, especially that of an ulcer surrounded by warty proliferations.

Involvement of mucosae, eye, nasal organs and bones is not uncommon on the face. Internal sporotrichosis is known, but is very rare, and may develop in any of the viscera.

Diagnosis. The disease must be distinguished from tuberculous, syphilitic and varicose ulceration. The so called 'fish tank granuloma' due to atypical mycobacteriae, especially *M. marinum*, may spread in a sporotrichoid manner on an arm. The diagnosis is made by histology and culture of biopsy material. Low temperature cultures are necessary to detect atypical mycobacteria.

Treatment. The prognosis is good if the disease is energetically treated. Potassium iodide should be given orally in full dosage for several weeks. The more serious forms of systemic sporotrichosis may respond to intravenous amphotericin B. There are conflicting reports concerning the use of griseofulvin in this infection. *Sporotrichum* is said not to be sensitive in vitro to this antibiotic, yet reports have been published claiming improvement and even cure of the lesions after several weeks' administration of the drug in the usual doses.

Maduramycosis (Madura foot)

This is a chronic granulomatous condition which affects the lower extremities, usually the foot. The disease is endemic in the tropical regions of Asia, Africa and America. It is mainly found amongst the bare-footed population of country districts and is an exogenous infection. It is caused by one of several different filamentous fungi including *Madurella* and *Nocardia* species. These fungi produce, in the diseased tissue, granules composed of hyphae and spores.

The tumour areas consist of granulation and fibrous tissue with abscess cavities and fistulae. The granules are found in the fluid in these cavities. There are three varieties of granules: white or yellow, brown or black, and red. They are 1 to 2 mm in diameter and irregular in shape and form. The presence of these granules confirms the diagnosis. The fasciae, muscles, tendons and bones are destroyed by the invasion of the fungus.

The fungi become lodged in small abrasions of the skin. Several months after the inoculation of the fungus, small hard nodules arise in the subcutaneous tissues. Ulceration occurs and a typical oily fluid which contains the granules is exuded. Other nodules form at the periphery, and in time the whole of the foot becomes involved. Necrosis of the bones occurs, and the foot is honeycombed with fistulae. The disease is not usually painful.

The prognosis depends on the causative organism. In resistant cases death occurs from cachexia or secondary infection.

Treatment. Prophylactic treatment consists in the adoption of adequate protection for the feet.

In early cases the nodules may be excised, but in the later stages amputation at some distance from the foot may be indicated. Nocardial infections (which have been said to account for 50% of cases in most districts) respond to sulphonamides, e.g. 6 – 8 g. sulphadiazine daily for many weeks. Penicillin or tetracycline, or even chloramphenicol should be given simultaneously. Madurellae are usually resistant to chemotherapy: di-amidinodiphenylamine, griseofulvin or amphotericin B may be tried.

Subcutaneous Phycomycosis

This is a subcutaneous eosinophilic granuloma due to *Basidiobolus meristosporus*, a fungus of the class Phycomycetes. The disease is usually seen in male children in the tropics but cases have been reported in England. It presents as firm, irregular, subcutaneous tumours, usually on the buttocks or thighs. Symptoms are minimal. Potassium iodide by mouth is the treatment of choice after the diagnosis has been established on biopsy material.

8

PARASITIC DISEASES

Scabies is a contagious disease due to *Sarcoptes scabiei hominis*, a tiny mite which burrows in the horny layer. The chief symptom is itching both at night and other times when the patient is warm. In the affected areas, vesicles, papules, pustules and burrows are found. The disease occurs in all classes of society and is spread by close and intimate contact, often within the family. Children may pass it from one to another in hand-holding games. Scabies may also be a venereal disease.

The female sarcoptes is about 400 μm in length and just visible to the naked eye (Fig. 39). The male is smaller. The fertilized female makes a burrow in the horny layer and remains there laying eggs which hatch in four days. Active larvae emerge and seek the shelter of hair follicles. The larvae moult becoming first nymphs and later adults. As adults they mate and the life cycle commences again. It takes about 17 days from egg to female adult.

Clinical picture. The distribution of the eruption is very characteristic, with lesions on some or all of the following sites: the webs of the fingers (Fig. 40), the flexor surfaces of the wrists, the elbows, the anterior and posterior axillary folds, round the umbilicus, the buttocks, the inner side of the thighs, the sides of the feet, the penis, around the nipples in women and on the palms and soles in infants. The burrows are thin sinuous lines on the skin from 1–10 mm in length. In a good light and with the aid of a lens, the sarcoptes can be seen at the closed end of their burrow as an oval glistening body with a brown or black dot at the front. The mite will adhere to a needle point inserted along the line of the burrow and can be placed on a slide and seen under the microscope.

Scabies is symptomless for the first month or two, then the host becomes sensitized to the mite and its products and itching

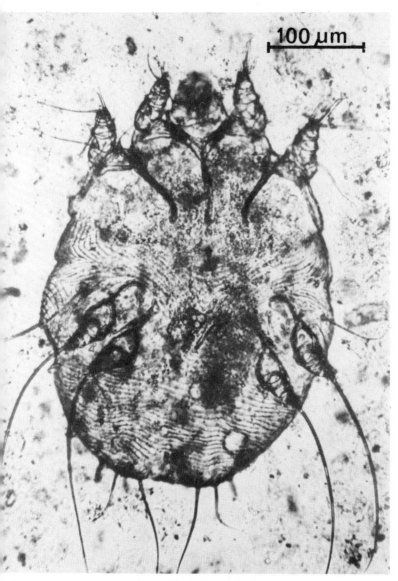

Fig. 39. Sarcoptes scabiei

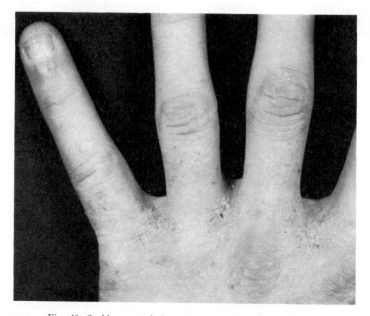

Fig. 40. Scabies: scratched papules and scaling between fingers.

develops. The irritation is most marked when the patient is warm e.g. in bed at night. It starts at the sites of infestation but may become so intense that it spreads to other sites and the whole body may become dermographic. In a second attack irritation starts immediately. Some individuals, mental defectives and those with poorly functioning brains are insensitive to itch stimuli and these people may develop huge colonies of sarcoptes with eczematous thickening of the skin. This condition, known as Norwegian scabies, is often unrecognized until there is an outbreak of scabies among the nurses, doctors and fellow patients of the source. In people who wash a lot it may be difficult or impossible to find a burrow and a therapeutic trial may be needed to make the diagnosis.

Eczematization and impetiginization may complicate scabies.

Treatment. It is desirable to treat all members of the patient's household and intimate contacts whether or not they have clinical scabies or symptoms. Failure to persuade the patient to consent to this is a common cause of recurrence. The patient and his contacts should take a bath at night time to soften the skin; after drying, 1% gamma benzene hexachloride cream (Lorexane, U.K.) or lotion (Quellada, U.K.; Kwell^R, U.S.A.) is applied all over the body up to the neck. The application is repeated after 24 hours and is finally washed off 48 hours after the start of the treatment. Special attention must be paid to the hands and feet, and the hands must be re-anointed after washing. There is no need to change the bed clothes or underclothing. Alternative treatments include benzyl benzoate B.P. application, which is effective but stings somewhat, and crotamiton (Eurax, U.K.) ointment or lotion which is so bland that it can be used for several days in succession. The lesions will not disappear immediately and a soothing application may be required, e.g. 1% hydrocortisone cream.

Secondary sepsis may also require attention. On the penis or trunk persistent indurated papules may remain for months and should be treated with a local steroid or crotamiton ointment.

Animal 'scabies'

Dogs may suffer from sarcoptic mange. Dogs, cats and rabbits may also be hosts to another species of mite, cheyletiella. These animal mites may produce papular urticaria with central necrosis of the papules, which is sometimes intensely itchy. The distribution in humans depends on the contacts with the animals. The finger webs and wrists tend not to be affected. Lesions occur on the arms, legs and trunk. The mites are small enough to penetrate clothing. The animals and the environment should be treated with appropriate insecticides; vacuum cleaning sucks up the eggs from the favoured chairs and the beds of the animals. Birds also have mites, e.g. budgerigars or birds that nest in the eaves of the house or in a broken air brick in a bed room. Chickens likewise have their own mite – *Dermanyssus gallinae*. Forage and grain may also be infested and produce papular urticaria.

FLEAS

Fleas produce an urticarial lesion with a central punctum (Fig. 41). The reaction is an immunological one so that if two individuals are bitten by the same flea, one may react briskly and the other not at all. The same may apply to other insects and is one reason

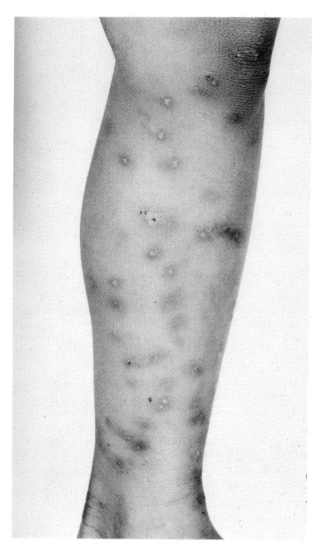

Fig. 41. Insect bites from the cat flea.

why only some members of the family have symptoms. Fleas may be of the human type or those of the cat, dog, rat, hedgehog or poultry. Fleas may remain viable up to 21 months away from the host and may be activated by vibration. The animal vector and the environment should be disinfected. The vacuum cleaner is useful for the latter.

BED BUGS

Bed bugs (*Cimex lenticularis*) measure 5 mm by 3 mm and live in walls, crevices, mattresses, ceilings and floors. Nocturnal in habit, they move with great agility and bite exposed parts, often producing a line of small weals with a central puncture. The local health authority should be called upon to disinfect dwellings. DDT or gamma benzene hexachloride in spray or powder are used.

An insect repellent such as diethyltoluamide gel or spray or diethyltoluamide and dimethylpthallate mixture as a liquid (Boots Co. Ltd., U.K.), is useful where it is impossible to control the environment. It should be applied to the exposed parts and renewed four-hourly. It is also especially useful out of doors against mosquitoes, midges and sandflies.

PEDICULOSIS

Pediculosis is an infestation of the hair or clothes with lice, which are wingless, blood-sucking insects. *Pediculus humanus* is 2–4 mm in length and lives on the scalp and body. *Pthirus pubis*, which is 1–2 mm in length and broad, is called the crab louse and lives in the public hair.

Pediculosis capitis

Pediculosis capitis is caused by *Pediculus humanus* var. *capitis*. It produces itching of the head and sometimes of the shoulders and regional lymphadenopathy. It is common in school children, especially those with long hair. The insects are difficult to find in clean school children but may be numerous in neglected adults (Fig. 42). The nits or egg cases can be seen readily in a good light. They are greyish white specks, 0.8 mm long, which are cemented to the hairs. They are laid at the scalp end of the hair and move out with the growth of the hair. They can sometimes be moved up and down the hair shaft but unlike scurf they are difficult to detach. Hair

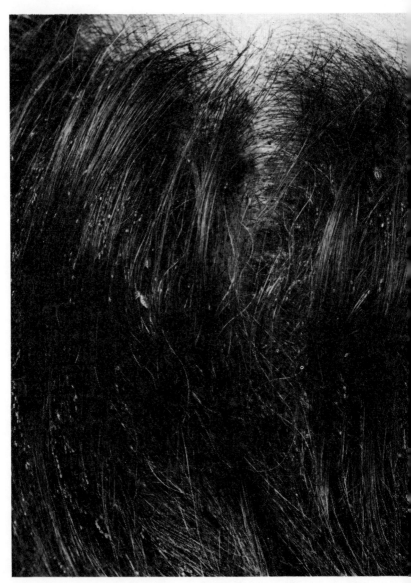

Fig. 42. Pediculosis capitis: a heavy infestation with nits and lice visible.

lacquer from a coarse spray can produce a passable imitation. Infection is passed by contact with an infected individual in the home, in schools and public transport, by combs, brushes and pillows. Secondary impetigo and lymphadenopathy are common complications.

Treatment. 1% gamma benzene hexachloride lotion (Quellada, U.K., Kwell^R, U.S.A.) is applied and left on for 24 hours. The treatment is repeated after one week because it is not effective against the ova. There is some evidence that head lice may become resistant to this drug and in such cases malathion 0.5% lotion (Prioderm Lotion, U.K.) is used instead. Empty egg cases are not a sign of continued infestation, and they may be removed with a nit comb. The inside of hats should be treated with gamma benzene hexachloride or dicophane (DDT) powder.

Pediculosis corporis

Pediculosis corporis is caused by *Pediculus humanus* var. *corporis* and occurs in tramps, vagrants and 'down and outs'. It causes widespread irritation, linear scratch marks on the back (Fig. 43),

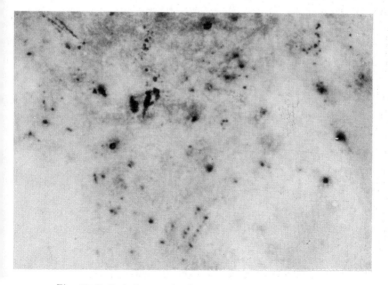

Fig. 43. Pediculosis corporis: linear scratch marks on the back.

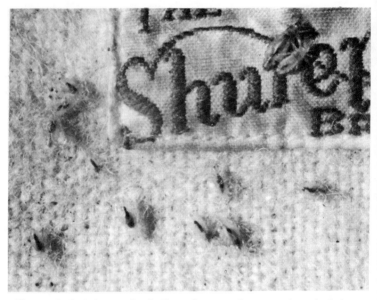

Fig. 44. Pediculosis corporis: the lice and eggs can be seen on the underclothes.

excoriations on the trunk and limbs and, in chronic infestations, pigmentation of the skin (vagabond's disease). The lice and the eggs are easily found in the seams of the clothes and underclothes rather than on the body (Fig. 44).

Treatment. The clothes and underclothes should be dusted with 10% dicophane (DDT) (B.P.C.) or 0.6% gamma benzene hexachloride powder (Insect and Louse Powder, ICI, U.K.). Alternatively, the clothes may be autoclaved.

Pediculosis pubis

Pediculosis pubis is caused by *Pthirus pubis* and affects the pubic and perineal hair. The nits can be seen and also sometimes the lice. Blue discoloured patches 0.2–3 cm in diameter, called maculae caeruleae, may be seen and are a reaction to material injected by the insect.

Treatment. Gamma benzene hydrochloride cream or lotion is applied twice at intervals of a week. If infestation is venereal in origin, other venereal diseases such as urethritis and lues should be excluded. If treatment fails, it is probably due to incorrect diagnosis, inadequate treatment or re-infection. *Pthirus pubis* is sometimes found on the eyelashes of a child, and can be treated by the application of 0.25% physostigmine eye drops to the actual insect.

9

CONTACT DERMATITIS

Contact dermatitis is a reaction to a substance in contact with the skin. The contact may be intentional or accidental. The causal substance may be obvious or it may require the ingenuity of a Sherlock Holmes to identify it. Careful notes and records should be kept, especially if the eczema is thought to be related to employment because occupational dermatitis of a non-infective nature caused by contact with dust, liquid, vapour or other irritants, qualifies for special payments under the National Insurance (Industrial Injuries) Act of the United Kingdom. The word dermatitis as used here is interchangeable with eczema but if the word dermatitis is used in the clinic the patient tends to regard the trouble as being caused by his work.

There are two main types of contact dermatitis, irritant contact dermatitis and allergic contact dermatitis. Other types are also seen.

IRRITANT DERMATITIS

Some substances are naturally irritating; solvents, surfactants, strong acids and alkalis are obvious examples. Petrol, paraffin and white spirit are also irritants and clothing soaked in any of these will produce erythema of thin skin within half an hour and, if the contact is prolonged, will produce blistering. These organic solvents are often used by people doing dirty, oily jobs to clean their hands. The skin of the palms is thick and there is no obvious effect at first but dermatitis may occur with prolonged, repeated use.

Strong soaps, detergents and moderately strong alkalis are used a great deal by housewives and it has been established that eczema of the hands is much commoner in women than in men (Figs. 45

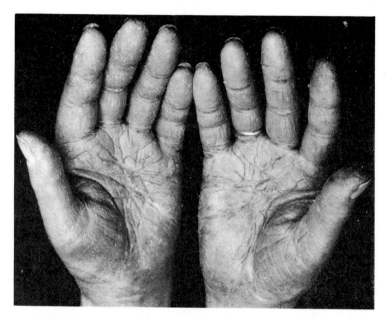

Fig. 45. Irritant dermatitis in a housewife.

and 46). Repeated chemical insults to the skin may be cumulative and produce permanent damage. Therefore, irritant dermatitis may be more difficult to cure than the allergic contact type. The hands are the commonest site and the reaction may be dryness, scaling with fissuring erythema and lichenification or, in acute episodes, erythema, vesiculation, blistering or even ulceration.

Prevention is much more efficacious than cure. Housewives should be encouraged to wear cotton lined plastic gloves for wet or dirty tasks and to use mops, tongs and washing machines. Workers in industry should be provided with gloves and protective clothing and, where possible, chemical processes should be mechanized. The provision of washing facilities is important. Barrier creams have little real barrier potential but they do enable chemical soil and dirt to be removed more easily. Irritants should be removed from the skin by vigorous washing in water and an emollient cream should be applied.

Allergic Contact Dermatitis

Allergic contact dermatitis is an immunological reaction and therefore does not occur until the body has become sensitized to a particular agent. Sensitization cannot take place in less than five days. The agents are usually non-irritant substances of a low molecular weight. Such a substance can penetrate the skin and, acting as a hapten, conjugate with a protein in the integument to form a complete antigen. This is conveyed to the regional lymph gland, possibly by the Langerhans cells. In the lymph gland the production of a special line of sensitized T-cells is initiated. Renewed contact with the agent will result in violent inflammation, the result of a reaction between the antigen and the sensitized T-lymphocytes. The reaction is of the delayed type IV kind. Circulating antibodies may also be produced and may be responsible for the spread of reactions by the formation of immune complexes. Although there is a minimum period before sensitization can occur, there is no maximum, hence substances which have been used by the patient for years should be viewed with a degree of suspicion, only slightly less than that of a new acquisition.

Some chemicals have an extraordinary capacity to excite sensitization. An example is DNCB (dinitrochlorobenzene), sensitization to which is regarded as a test of the patient's ability to produce a normal cell-mediated immune response.

Medicaments

Bitter experience has taught us that certain drugs should not be used as local applications on the skin because they have a high sensitization potential. Penicillin, streptomycin, sulphonamides, local anaesthetics of the procaine series and antihistamines should never be used as topical applications. Neomycin is a sensitizer but penetrates the intact horny layer poorly and may be used in ointments, creams and lotions. It is unwise to use it or its analogue soframycin in the treatment of long standing eczema or leg ulcers, which are by nature chronic, because the prolonged exposure is likely to lead to sensitization over the years.

Creams and lotions contain preservatives such as parabens or chlorocresol. These are put in to prevent bacteria or fungi growing but they do produce sensitization. Surprisingly, lanolin in ointments, creams and lotions may produce sensitization too. Doctors

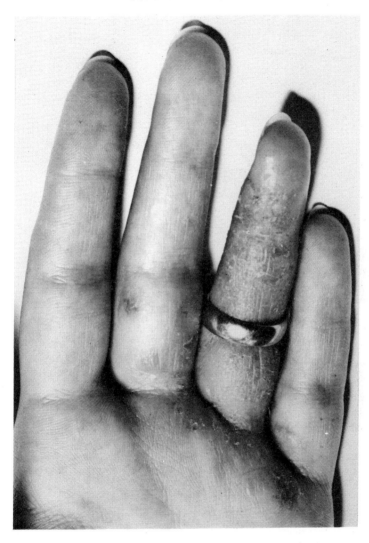

Fig. 46. Irritant dermatitis due to soap and washing powder trapped under a ring. Tests for metals allergies were negative.

and nurses may be in contact with penicillin, streptomycin, chlor-promazine (Largactil, Thorazine, U.K.), local anaesthetics, anti-septics, formalin, glutaraldehyde and rubber gloves which can all sensitize the skin. Dentists additionally are in contact with acrylic resins used for dentures and essential oils such as eugenol, oil of cloves and Balsam of Peru.

Cosmetics

Cosmetics cause dermatitis relatively rarely. Face and other creams may contain lanolin and preservatives, and perfumes themselves or as an ingredient of other toilet preparations may produce reactions. Hair dyes, which contain *para*phenylene or *para*toluene diamine, produce less trouble now than formerly, presumably because of refinement of the application technique. Dermatitis caused by hair dyes presents as itching round the hair margin and ears and oedema of the eyelids. The dermatitis of the scalp itself may be late in appearing and mild in degree because this region is resistant and relatively unreactive. Lipstick some-times produces allergic cheilitis, usually caused by the eosin con-stituent. Nail varnish reactions are remarkable because the nails themselves seldom show reactions, being made of hard, dead keratin; more often it is the areas of skin touched by the nails which show inflammation and itching, e.g. the neck, chin and eyelids (Fig. 47).

Clothing

Clothing also produces relatively little in the way of problems. Wool does not induce allergy although its barbed fibres will irritate a sensitive skin. Nylon and other synthetic fibres are made of large insoluble molecules which are unreactive. Dyes may occasionally become leached from fabrics and produce 'nylon stocking der-matitis' or eruptions on the body and arms.

Metals

Nickel sensitivity is common in women although less so now than in the days of suspenders (garters). Zip fasteners, earrings, rings, bracelets, necklaces, watches, watch straps, and brassiere clips may all produce reactions (Fig. 48). Cobalt is often a contaminant of nickel and allergy to both metals is common. This is of impor-tance in those about to receive total hip replacement and other

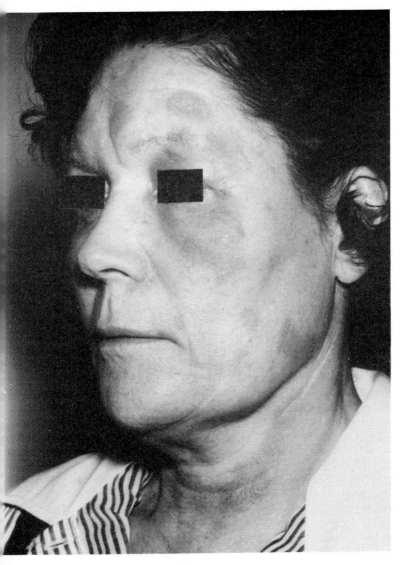

Fig. 47. Nail varnish dermatitis: the eyelids are red and swollen and there is erythema on the face and neck. The nails and fingers were unaffected.

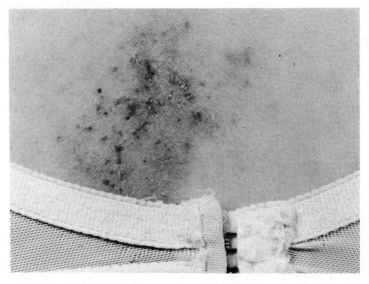

Fig. 48. Metal dermatitis caused by a nickel-plated brassiere fastener.

prostheses. Chromium sensitivity is commoner in men than women. Building workers with eczema of the hands and arms are often allergic to chromium which is present in some cements. Chromates are also used to tan leather and have a wide variety of uses in industry.

Rubber

Natural latex as it comes from the tree is harmless but when it is processed, accelerators and antioxidants are added, some of which are powerful sensitizers. Rubber gloves, the rubber in brassieres and other under garments, rubber wellington boots, rubber shoe soles, rubber bands and condoms may produce reactions (Fig. 50).

Plastics

Plastic objects in the home rarely cause trouble because the plastic is in the polymerized state. Acrylic monomer occasionally pro duces trouble in dentists and dental technicians, because it penetrates rubber gloves easily. Acrylic monomer has produced eczema of the hands in an orthopaedic surgeon. Light-sensitive acrylates are used to produce ink and plates in new printing technology and have caused outbreaks of dermatitis. Epoxy and other resins are widely used in industry, in the home as 'Araldite' glue and as plastic material for mending car body work and for making boats; both the resins and their separate hardeners are allergenic.

Plants

Plants should always be considered in the diagnosis of eczematous conditions. In England the treacherous *Primula obconica* is treasured in many an unsuspecting home. It contains a powerful sensitizer and often produces linear blisters or erythemas on the exposed parts of the face, arms and hands (Fig. 52). Chrysanthemums are fairly potent sensitizers and the amateur or professional gardener or the flower shop worker is at risk. Tulip bulb and garlic clove

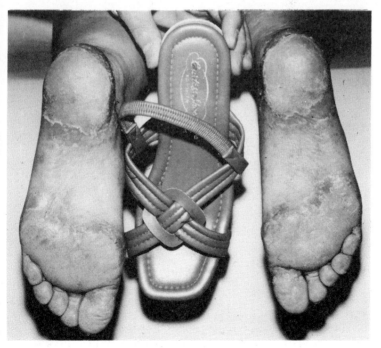

Fig. 49. Sandal dermatitis.

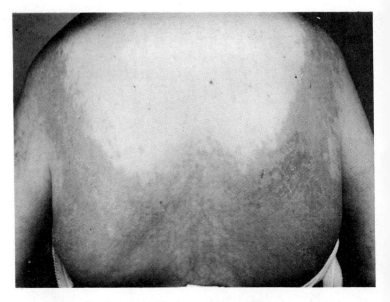

Fig. 50. Brassiere dermatitis from a rubber stabilizer in a garment.

allergies result in fissured dermatitis of the finger tips. In North America and Asia, poison oak and ivy produce substantial morbidity. Wood dermatitis occurs mainly in those who work with wood; teak, teak substitutes and other exotic aromatic woods are known allergens.

CLINICAL PICTURE

The skin itches and develops redness, swelling, vesication and scaling. The site is usually the part exposed to the allergen. However, the nails and thickly keratinized palms and soles may not react, but transfer the allergen, causing the rash to appear elsewhere. The eyelids, the antecubital fossae, the penis and scrotum are often secondary sites. Great oedema of the soft parts such as the eyelids and the scrotum is often a feature. The oedema is followed by blistering or scaling unlike angio-oedema (Plate VIII).

The exposed parts and the sides and backs of the fingers and hands are the most commonly affected areas.

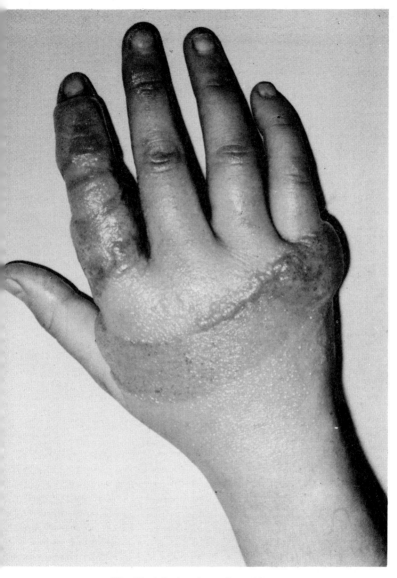

Fig. 51. Adhesive plaster dermatitis.

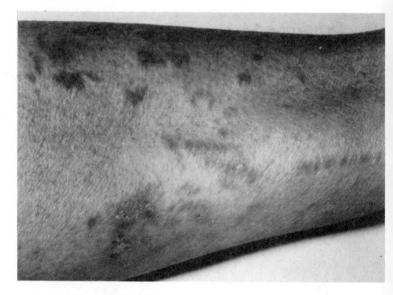

Fig. 52. Primula and chrysanthemum dermatitis. Note linear streaks on arms.

DIAGNOSIS

Diagnosis depends on detective work. It may be easy if the condition is intermittent and corresponds to an unusual activity. The history is of great importance. It is useful to list what substances the patient encounters, whether new or old, in the home, at work and in the pursuit of hobbies or sports.

Patch testing

Patch testing is the controlled application of possible allergens to the skin and is the most useful technique for investigating allergic contact dermatitis. It is of no use in irritant dermatitis, because every irritant will produce a positive reaction, and of little use in urticaria or drug eruptions. The test substances must be diluted to an appropriate strength in petroleum jelly, water, acetone or olive oil. A small amount is placed on a little square of cloth on a piece of polythene. The patch is put on the back and kept in place with zinc oxide strapping. It is removed and read at 48 hours and four days. A positive response varies in intensity from erythema, via vesica-

TABLE II. The International Contact Dermatitis Research Group Standard Battery of Patch Test Substances.

	Test Substance	Concentration %
0001	potassium dichromate	0.5
0002	cobalt chloride	1
0003	nickel sulphate	5
0004	formaldehyde (in water)	1
0005	paraphenylenediamine (PPD)	2
0008	balsam of Peru	25
0009	turpentine peroxides (in olive oil)	0.3
0010	neomycin sulphate	20
0012	parabens (methyl-, ethyl-, propyl-, butyl-, benzyl; 3% of each)	15
0015	chinoform	5
0017	colophony	20
0019	wood tars (pine, beech, juniper, birch; 3% of each)	12
0020	wool alcohols	30
0021	epoxy resin	1
0022	mercaptomix	2
0023	thiuram-mix	1
0024	PPD-mix	0.6
0025	naphthyl-mix	1
0026	carbamix	3
0027	ethylene diamine	2
0028	cinnamaldehyde	2

0022, 0023, 0024, 0025, 0026 are rubber additives.

These materials may be obtained from: Karen Trolle-Lassen, 6B, A.N. Hansens Alle, 2900, Hellerup, Denmark.

tion to bulla formation and even ulceration. A control patch is applied in case there is a reaction to the plaster. The substances used for testing are those used by the patient. Most dermatological centres with a special interest in the subject will also apply a standard battery of contact allergens (Table II) based on the recommendations of the International Contact Dermatitis Research Group. It basically includes nickel, cobalt and chromium salts, rubber compounds, hair dye, local anaesthetics and resins. The battery test may alert the physician to the possibility of contracts not discovered in the history.

Sometimes it is impossible to arrange a patch test. In such a case the patient should be advised to avoid likely allergens and if improvement occurs to reintroduce contact to the suspected substances one by one.

TREATMENT

If possible the cause should be identified and removed.

Acute reactions

If there are blisters these should be pricked after cleaning the skin with potassium permanganate, 1:5,000 in water. Wet dressings of normal saline or aluminium acetate (Burow's solution) may be applied or a steroid ointment or cream used four times a day. If the reaction is very severe it is justifiable to administer a short course of steroids: prednisone 30 to 40 mg a day for seven days reducing the dose slowly to zero over the next 7 – 10 days, or a single injection of 40 to 80 mg of methyl prednisolone acetate (Depo-Medrone, U.K.; Depo-Medrol℞, U.S.A.).

Subacute and chronic reactions

Subacute and chronic reactions are treated with potassium permanganate, 1:5000, soaks, followed by the application of a strong steroid ointment or cream, which is continued in a diluted form (1 in 5 or 1 in 10) twice a day (see Appendix). Secondary infection should be treated with a local antiseptic or antibiotic incorporated in the local steroid or by systemic administration. Antihistamines may be given for itching but the patient should be warned about the sedative side effects, especially if they drive or work with machinery. Sedation at night with nitrazepam, 5 mg, may also be required. If the hands are affected they should be treated with great respect for a long time after recovery; cotton-lined plastic gloves should be worn for wet and dirty tasks. Irritant dermatitis is treated in the same way but systemic steroids are seldom indicated.

OTHER TYPES OF CONTACT REACTION

Some substances sensitize the skin to light, e.g. meadow grass, parsnips and the bergamot oil in eau de cologne and perfumes.

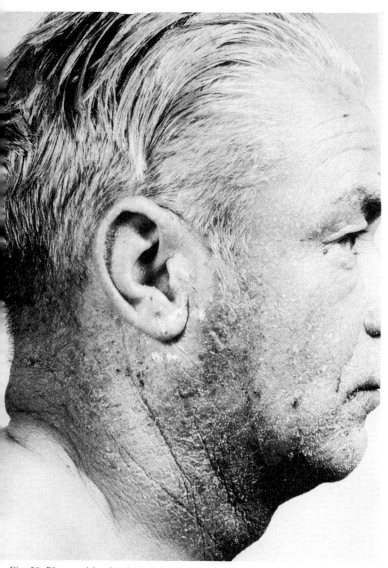

Fig. 53. Photosensitization dermatitis caused by antiseptic soap. Note sharp cut-off at collar.

This is a phototoxic reaction. Other compounds are activated by light and produce allergic reactions, e.g. chlorpromazine, promethazine and the antiseptics bithionol and tetrachlorsalicylanilide which have been used in toilet articles, soap, tooth paste and hair creams (Fig. 53). Machine oil and tar can produce folliculitis of the hairy areas of the trunk, limbs and face. Halogenated phenols may produce severe acne, not only on the areas contaminated but also on other areas of the body. Tar, asphalt, pitch and mineral oil especially in combination with light can produce pigmentation, telangiectasia, degeneration of the skin and later keratoses and cancer. Repeated injury, trauma and abrasion in building workers and miners may produce permanent damage to the skin.

10

ECZEMA

Eczema is a non-infective inflammatory disorder of the skin. It should be regarded as a 'reaction pattern' rather than a specific disease and can have many external and internal causes. Genetic, immunological, infective, vascular, traumatic and emotional factors may all play a part at different times in the causation of endogenous eczema. The word 'eczema' has a Greek derivation meaning 'to flow out' and implies an exudative eruption. In this book, 'eczema' is synonymous with 'dermatitis' and 'eczematous dermatitis'. Externally caused eczema (contact dermatitis) is discussed in the previous chapter. Here, internal or endogenous eczema is described.

Pathology

Eczema affects the upper dermis and epidermis. The initial change is extra- and intra-cellular oedema of the lower epidermis, known as spongiosis. The prickle cells swell and separate until microscopic vesicles form. Epidermal maturation is disturbed by unknown factors and epidermal thickening or acanthosis, hyperkeratosis and parakeratosis result. As the vesicles enlarge they involve the superficial epidermis and become visible. As the roofs of vesicles are rubbed off, exudation follows, encouraged by the leakage of oedema fluid from the spongiotic epidermis. Exudation may be followed by crust formation. In the dermis, the capillaries and lymphatics are dilated and an infiltrate of white cells accumulates, which is mainly lymphocytic but has some polymorphonuclear leucocytes. Some of these cells migrate into the epidermis.

In chronic eczema, the epidermis progressively thickens, partly due to rubbing. Spongiosis persists but vesicles are no longer seen. The dermal infiltrate becomes more pleomorphic.

Symptoms and signs

The symptoms of eczema are itching, often intense, and the development of a vesicular, then 'weeping' rash. Examination reveals a zone of erythema and oedema. In acute eczema, uniformly distributed pinhead to match-head sized vesicles are seen in the inflamed area. In sub-acute eczema, the vesicles are less prominent and thickening of the skin, scaliness, fissuring and crusting ensue. In the chronic stage, the oedematous, parakeratotic, thickened epidermis has a characteristic appearance and 'feel', with exaggerated skin lines. This condition is called lichenification. Eczema always itches and the pruritus may be evident in scratch marks and the burnished surfaces of the finger nails.

Course, spread and prognosis

The course of all patterns of eczema is enormously variable and unpredictable. Its changes are reversible and resolved eczema leaves no permanent scarring or other evidence of its presence.

Active eczema often has a tendency to spread from its initial site and may do so by direct extension, indirect extension (neighbouring but not contiguous lesions), contralateral imitation or widespread symmetrical outbreaks.

Lichenification and prurigo are common complications of eczema. Secondary infection may be obvious or covert, taking the form of impetiginization, folliculitis or even boils.

Classification

Classification of eczema is arbitrary and is based on the principal patterns observed in practice. The following types may be seen.
1. Atopic eczema.
2. Seborrhoeic eczema (including otitis externa and intertrigo).
3. Hypostatic (varicose) eczema.
4. Nummular (discoid) eczema.
5. Pompholyx.
6. Asteatotic eczema.
7. Neurodermatitis (lichen simplex chronicus).
8. Prurigo.
9. Infective eczematoid dermatitis.
10. Generalized exfoliative dermatitis.
11. Miscellaneous.

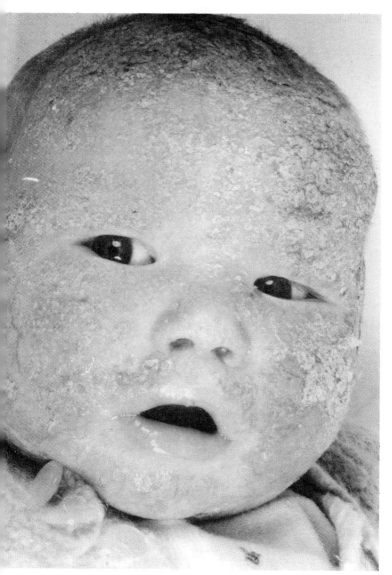

Fig. 54. Severe atopic eczema in an infant.

ATOPIC ECZEMA

This is a pattern of chronic eczema which usually begins in childhood and is sometimes associated with bronchial asthma, hay fever, vernal conjunctivitis or urticaria. Other associated conditions may include a dry skin, a tendency to increased cutaneous vasoconstrictor tone and rare eye defects, namely juvenile cataract and keratoconus. There is often a family history of some of these conditions.

The eczema typically begins in the third or fourth month of life as a symmetrically distributed eruption on the forehead, cheeks, trunks and limbs (Fig. 54). The affected areas are red, exudative and crusted and the child scratches when given the opportunity. At the toddler stage, the eczema increasingly involves the limb flexures and becomes lichenified (Figs 55 and 56).

The course is exceedingly variable. Atopic eczema may be a transient problem of infancy or may be a debilitating life-long disease. It often remits in middle childhood only to recur in early adult life but in 90% of subjects the condition has apparently cleared by puberty. Atopic eczema may begin in adolescence or even in adult life, when papular or nodular lichenification (prurigo) is common (Fig. 57).

Asthma, hay fever and urticaria, which can be associated with atopic eczema, appear later in childhood. They may be transient or chronic and may be provoked by specific inhalants or ingestants. The increased vasoconstrictor tone is one manifestation of a little understood disorder of cutaneous blood vessels and is responsible for the characteristic 'muddy' pallor of the severe atopic. It can be demonstrated as a paradoxical vasoconstrictor response to stimuli which are normally vasodilatory, e.g. firm stroking of the skin (white dermographism) or the intra-cutaneous injection of carbachol (delayed blanch phenomenon).

Hay fever, vernal conjunctivitis, urticaria and possibly asthma are apparently the result of an immune disorder characterized by an enhanced liability to develop Type I (reaginic) antibodies. These are apparent as excess serum IgE immunoglobulins, which are formed in response to many common inhaled and ingested allergens. The presence of specific IgE antibodies can be demonstrated crudely by intradermal or 'prick' testing and, in the laboratory, by immuno-assay techniques with specific antigens. Anaphylactic reactions to drugs, especially penicillin and antisera, are a hazard.

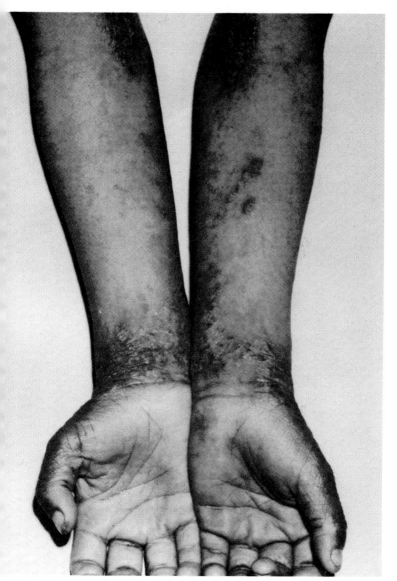

Fig. 55. Atopic eczema: lichenified flexure.

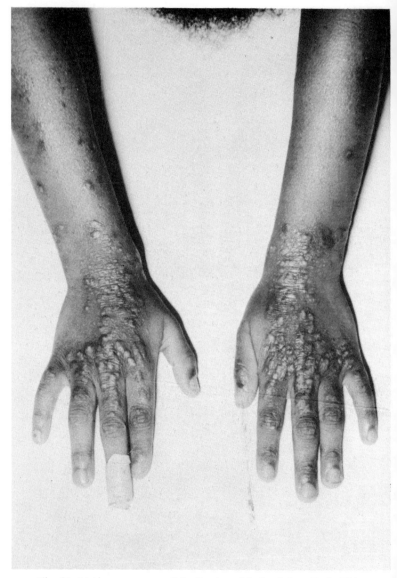

Fig. 56. Atopic eczema: gross lichenification of the hands in a black child.

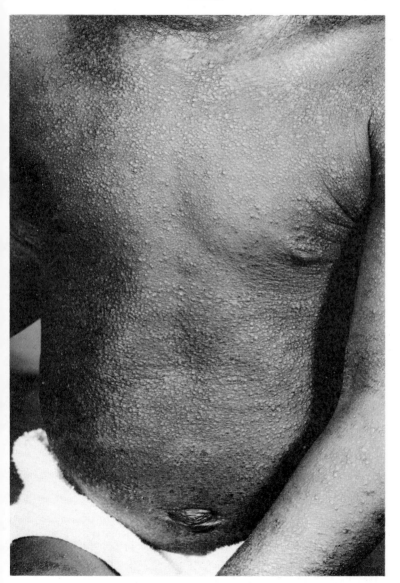

Fig. 57. Atopic eczema: profuse papular lichenification in a black child.

The dry skin (xeroderma, ichthyosis), found in 20% of atopic subjects, is probably due to an associated genetic defect. Atopics do not have any increased liability to develop allergic contact dermatitis but their threshold for irritant contact dermatitis, e.g. from detergents, is lowered. They are not particularly vulnerable to secondary bacterial infection of the skin, although such impetiginization is sometimes seen (Fig. 58). They are, however, particularly vulnerable to primary infection with herpes simplex and vaccinia viruses. These infections, eczema herpeticum or eczema vaccinatum (Fig. 59), may cause a severe viral pyoderma with fever and may be fatal. Both were originally described as Kaposi's varicelliform eruption. In addition, viral warts and the lesions of molluscum contagiosum may sometimes be very numerous in atopic subjects. Interestingly, other viral infections such as measles, varicella and rubella behave normally.

The cause of atopic eczema is not understood. Genetic factors are obviously important but the precise mode of inheritance is unknown. Recent work has shown that atopic babies have extremely low secretory IgA levels for several months. Since this is the immunoglobulin which protects epithelial surfaces, it has been suggested that during this period potentially antigenic inhalants and ingestants enter the body in large amounts, stimulating the formation of IgE reaginic antibodies. However, although it is clear that the asthma, hay fever and urticaria of atopy are due to these immune disturbances, it is by no means established that the eczema is similarly explained.

SEBORRHOEIC ECZEMA

This name is unfortunate since the patterns of eczema so labelled are unrelated to seborrhoea (excessive sebum production), but no better term has gained acceptance. The following patterns can be seen.

An eruption of the scalp, which can spread to the ears, neck and face, may present as a superficial branny scaling causing dandruff or a more severe eczema with exudation, crusting or thick scales. The latter type may spread to the ears and eyebrows and beyond to the trunk and main body folds as an 'exudative' and often infected eczema (see Fig. 11).

The midline of the chest pre-sternally and between the shoulder

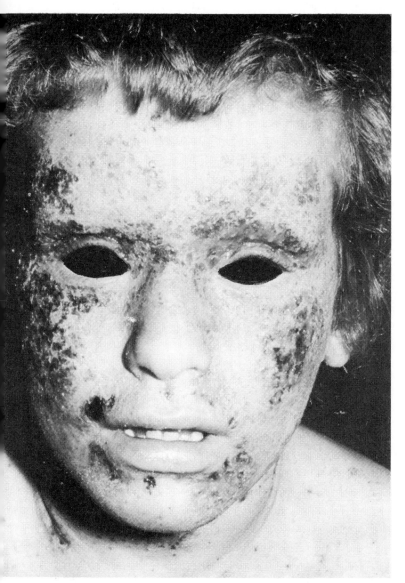

Fig. 58. Impetiginized atopic eczema in an older boy.

blades may show a chronic yellowish red petaloid rash. Itching is very variable and the surface is greasy rather than scaly. The skin around the nose may be similarly involved and sometimes the brow.

These patients are prone to coccal infections. Chronic blepharitis, folliculitis, especially of the beard, and 'boils' are common and cocci are easily cultured from lesions not obviously infected.

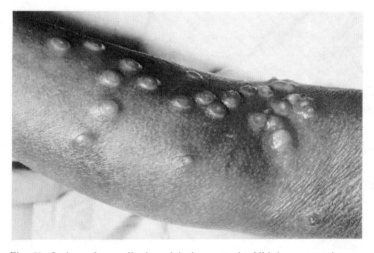

Fig. 59. Lesions of generalized vaccinia in an atopic child (eczema vaccinatum, Kaposi's varicelliform eruption). Note umbilication of lesions.

Chronic otitis externa

This pattern of seborrhoeic eczema is probably provoked by infective, climatic or chemical factors. Infection derived from the middle ear should be obvious and distinguishable from the spectrum of Gram-positive or Gram-negative secondary bacterial invaders. The entities of 'desert ear' and 'swimming pool ear' testify to the importance of excessive climatic dryness and wetness respectively. Chemical factors are secondary but may be important in perpetuating the condition. Sensitization by nickel hair pins, phosphorous sesquisulphide from red headed matches, or the constituents of creams and ointments is not uncommon.

Intertrigo

Eczema may occur at the sites of skin folds, e.g. under the breasts, in the abdominal folds of the obese and in the ano-genital areas. Increased humidity and warmth encourage bacterial or yeast proliferation and friction, hyperhidrosis and scratching may be added factors. A variety of micro-organisms is always found but the condition is rarely purely infective and can be regarded as a pattern of seborrhoeic eczema.

It is convenient to consider pruritus ani and pruritus vulvae here although these conditions may not have an eczematous basis.

PRURITUS ANI

Pruritus ani is a common symptom. In childhood it is usually due to threadworm infestation. In adult life it almost always affects men. It may be transient or chronic and has many causes. Infective causes include viral warts, candidiasis (e.g. after wide-spectrum oral antibiotic therapy), erythrasma and in rare cases tinea. Bacterial infection also plays a role in seborrhoeic intertrigo where there is usually also an eczematous factor. Other forms of eczema which may be responsible are contact dermatitis medicamentosa and neurodermatitis. Other skin diseases, such as psoriasis and lichen planus, may involve the peri-anal skin and present as pruritus ani. Surgical causes include fistula, fissure-in-ano, haemorrhoids and skin tags. Any rectal discharge may cause pruritus so that occasionally a carcinoma of the rectum, gonococcal proctitis, rectal incontinence or excessive use of liquid paraffin as a laxative may be responsible.

Notwithstanding this long list of established causes, pruritus ani may occur in the absence of any of them and may persist or be intermittent for decades. Obesity, a tendency to hyperhidrosis in the ano-genital area, poor hygiene after defaecation, especially in the hirsute, and imperceptible leakage of rectal mucus on to the peri-anal skin may each be relevant. In the past, when no physical cause of such an intractable symptom could be found, psychosexual explanations found particular favour. It is true that many men with this symptom readily, and apparently with a complete lack of natural modesty, present the offending orifice for examination by the doctor; an observation which has been cited as evidence of latent or suppressed homosexuality. They may also display a good deal of anxiety in various ways. Nevertheless, the authors remain unconvinced by the evidence adduced in favour of psychogenic mechanisms, although their importance in a small minority of patients cannot be denied.

Whatever the cause, the physical signs vary from slight erythema to excoriation, lichenification, and secondary folliculitis. In all cases, examination must be thorough and should include digital rectal examination, proctoscopy and Wood's light examination of the peri-anal skin. If no treatable surgical or dermatological entity is found, management should include attention to bowel habit and hygiene after defaecation. Cleansing the area after defaecation with soap and water rather than toilet paper may be helpful. Hydrocortisone ointment 1% may be useful, as may a preparation combining hydrocortisone with lignocaine (Xyloproct ointment, U.K.).

Pruritus Vulvae

This is a common symptom which may present to the general practitioner, gynaecologist or dermatologist. Usually a physical explanation can be found. The important causes are:

1. Vaginal discharge, whether trichomonal or candidial or due to cervicitis.

2. Urinary incontinence or glycosuria.

3. Local skin disease such as pediculosis pubis, psoriasis, eczema of various types, senile atrophy, lichen sclerosus et atrophicus or leukoplakia.

As in men with pruritus ani, obesity and poor hygiene may increase the liability to intertrigo. Possibly the replacement of stockings by occlusive tights has also been an aggravating factor in some cases. When no physical cause is apparent, psychosexual explanations have been invoked but are hard to establish.

Treatment depends on the cause. In idiopathic cases, weak topical corticosteroid creams such as 1% hydrocortisone cream are useful. Oestrogen cream has a place in the management of senile atrophy.

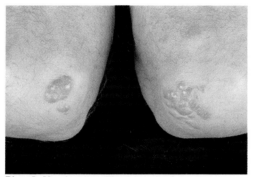

Plate I. Xanthomata. The colour is often more yellow and orange than shown on the illustration.

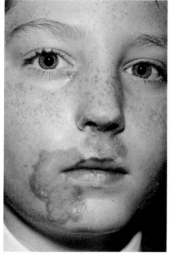

Plate II. Impetigo.

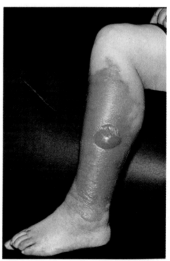

Plate III. Erysipelas. Note the sharp margins.

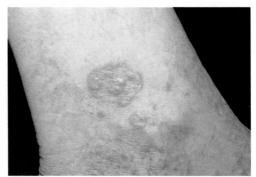

Plate IV. Lichen planus.

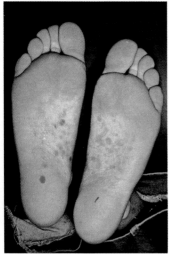

Plate V. Secondary syphilis: maculopapular lesions.

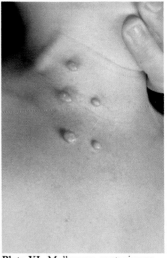

Plate VI. Molluscum contagiosum. Note the umbilication.

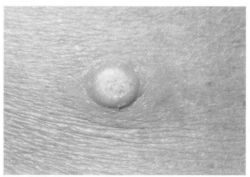

Plate VII. Keratoacanthoma: convex border with central keratinization.

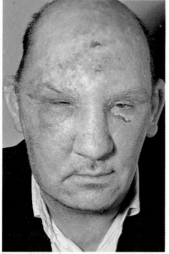

Plate VIII. Contact dermatitis. Note the scaling and the oedema of the eyelids.

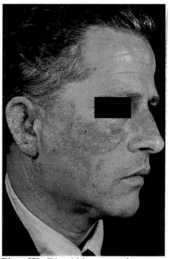

Plate IX. Discoid lupus erythematosus.

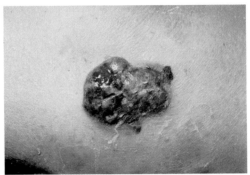

Plate X. Malignant melanoma, showing irregularity of colour and contour.

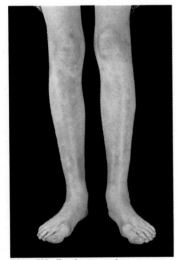

Plate XI. Erythema nodosum.

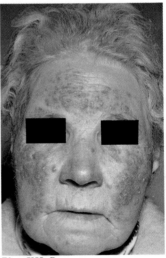

Plate XII. Rosacea.

HYPOSTATIC ECZEMA

Also called gravitational, varicose or venous eczema, hypostatic eczema is one of the common clinical manifestations of chronic venous insufficiency in the leg. The other features of the syndrome include oedema, induration, varicosities, purpura, brown pigmentation due to haemosiderin staining of the skin, ulceration and areas of replacement of the skin by scar tissue called 'white atrophy'.

The eczema usually begins as an irregular area of erythema followed by scaling and later exudation and crusting. It is seen on the lower third of the calf and about the malleoli (Fig. 60). It tends

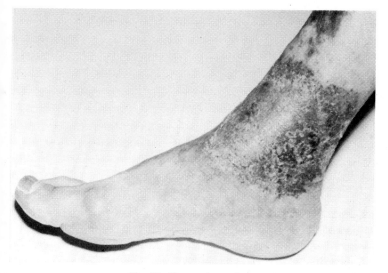

Fig. 60. Hypostatic eczema.

to spread slowly especially if the underlying oedema is not controlled. This type of eczema has a particular tendency to disseminate widely and is often complicated by an allergic contact dermatitis due to topically applied medications (see p. 112). It may also be complicated by episodes of erysipelas, cellulitis and superficial phlebitis, especially if it is associated with an ulcer. These episodes may be followed by chronic organized oedema.

NUMMULAR (DISCOID) ECZEMA

This is a little understood pattern of endogenous eczema in adults characterized by the appearance of multiple well defined discoid lesions, usually on the limbs but sometimes on the trunk. The lesions tend to recur at the same sites, sometimes over years. Nummular eczema sometimes seems to be precipitated by emotional stress in men in the late middle years but usually no cause is obvious.

Nummular eczema may also occur in persons with atopic eczema and also in those with contact dermatitis. The eczema of the nipples and areolae which occurs in young women resembles nummular eczema but the causation remains uncertain apart from a minority with definite atopic disease.

POMPHOLYX

It is traditional to use this term for a singular idiopathic pattern of eczema of the palms (cheiropompholyx) and soles (podopompholyx). Afflicted individuals are prone to recurrent attacks of eczema at one or both of these sites, particularly in spring and summer. Itching and redness are associated with the formation of tiny vesicles along the sides of fingers and on the palms or soles which may appear in crops and persist for weeks or months. Rarely, attacks are fulminating and the vesicles run together to form huge blisters which may become secondarily infected by streptococci and staphylococci. Such attacks may be totally disabling and subsequent peeling of the lifted-off stratum corneum 'de-gloves' the extremities.

Again, as with nummular eczema, the clinician must be aware that vesicular palmo-plantar eczema may have a precise cause. It may be a manifestation of a contact dermatitis or it may be secondary to contact dermatitis elsewhere on the body, e.g. rubber dermatitis of the feet or neomycin dermatitis around a varicose ulcer. Rarely, it may be caused by an acute inflammatory tinea pedis. It is thus inappropriate to label all vesicular palmo-plantar eczema as pompholyx.

ASTEATOTIC ECZEMA

With advancing age, a singular pattern of eczema is often seen, particularly on the shins. It consists of modest erythema, fine

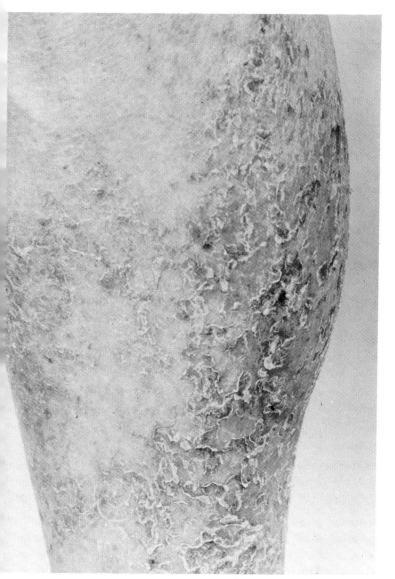

Fig. 61. Asteatotic eczema (eczéma cracquelé).

scaling and very superficial 'crazy pavement' fissuring which combine to produce a characteristic pattern, sometimes called 'eczéma cracquelé' (Fig. 61). Asteatotic eczema is common in old people with inadequately heated homes when the weather is cold and dry and may be encouraged by hypothyroidism and therapy with powerful diuretics.

NEURODERMATITIS

The term 'neurodermatitis' is as confusing as 'seborrhoeic'. In the authors' opinion, the term should be reserved for the peculiar, localized lichenification, lichen simplex chronicus. This type of skin disorder is seen mostly in adult women, particularly on the occipital scalp, nape, sides of the neck, high on the ulnar forearm near the elbow, volar wrist, sides of the lower calves and sides of the natal cleft. Chronic pruritus ani and pruritus vulvae may lead to localized lesions.

The lesions are sharply defined, raised plaques and often ovoid or elongated. Hyperpigmentation is common and the surface shows exaggerated skin markings. The yellow/brown races are particularly susceptible to this pattern and to lichenification in general.

Itching is intermittent and intense and patients usually admit that they habitually rub the lesions, particularly when agitated. These patients commonly reveal evidence of emotional stresses so that retention of the term 'neurodermatitis' seems justified.

It should be mentioned that the term disseminated neurodermatitis is often used for generalized atopic eczema in the United States.

PRURIGO

This is yet another confusing and ambiguous term. It should be reserved for a papular or nodular eruption which itches intensely and which is partly a pattern of lichenification perpetuated by rubbing or pinching the skin. The histology is eczematous. These lesions are often widely scattered on the trunk and limbs.

Prurigo may be part of the atopic spectrum or be reproduced by insect bites. It may prove to be a manifestation of a lympho-reticular malignancy or renal failure. Some prurigo is certainly psychogenic but exclusion of underlying organic causes is mandatory before the condition is classified as psychogenic or idiopathic in origin.

INFECTIVE ECZEMATOID DERMATITIS

This term is applied to an uncommon localized pattern of eczema, usually seen on the hands, in which centrifugally spreading eczema is evidently associated with local infection. The pattern is often preceded by minor physical or chemical traumas, particularly in an industrial setting.

GENERALIZED EXFOLIATIVE DERMATITIS

This is a distinct syndrome, also called erythroderma, in which the skin is universally inflamed, red, oedematous and scaly (Fig. 62), submerging any localized lesions, although it is not always eczematous. The course may be sub-acute or chronic but eventual spontaneous remission is usual.

Most cases of eczematous generalized exfoliative dermatitis arise for unknown reasons from unclassified eczema of the head and neck or extremities, often within a few weeks of onset. Erythroderma may be caused by psoriasis, pityriasis rubra pilaris (a rare entity of unknown cause), drugs such as barbiturates, phenylbutazone, P.A.S. and gold, lymphomas and leukaemias. Less often injudicious topical therapy, or persistent exposure to an unrecognized antigen, is responsible.

Exfoliative dermatitis may be complicated by extreme thickening and deep fissuring of the palms and soles, gross nail dystrophy, loss of head and body hair (reversible) and superficial lymphadenopathy (dermatopathic lymphadenitis). The metabolic sequelae are described on p. 195.

MISCELLANEOUS

Drug eruptions may be eczematous (see above). Rarely metabolic disorders are associated with eczema, e.g. phenylketonuria in infants, Wiskott-Aldrich syndrome, steatorrhoea and Danbolt's acrodermatitis enteropathica. Congenital lymphatic dysplasias may predispose to eczema in the lower leg. Polymorphic light eruption is an eczema of the exposed parts occurring in spring and summer; the patient may react abnormally to short wave ultraviolet light and longer wavelengths.

gitis and lymphadenitis or cellulitis. The responsible organism is usually *Streptococcus pyogenes* and penicillin is the drug of choice. Mixed staphylococcal and streptococcal infections may fail to respond to penicillin, in which case a change to erythromycin or flucloxacillin is indicated.

Staphylococcal folliculitis and 'boils', sometimes attributable to topical steroids, may be a second indication for the systemic use of antibiotics. Choice of antibiotic should be guided by bacteriological sensitivities. A third indication is infected seborrhoeic dermatitis.

Antihistamines may be of limited value in allaying itching and encouraging sleep. Psychotropic drugs may also have a limited place especially in atopic eczema and neurodermatitis in adults.

In certain circumstances, oral steroid therapy does have a place in the treatment of eczema. Prednisolone 30 – 40 mg daily may be invaluable if used early in a fulminating attack of pompholyx. A similar dosage is used in generalized exfoliative dermatitis, especially if dangerous metabolic sequelae are threatening (see p. 196).

Much lower dosages of prednisolone, i.e. 5 – 10 mg daily, have a place in the long-term management of resistant and disabling extensive chronic eczema of any type. Alternatively, weekly or twice weekly injections of tetracosactrin zinc (Synacthen Depot, U.K.) can be used.

11

DRUG ERUPTIONS

Drug reactions are extremely common and their diversity has led to their replacing the last century's syphilis and tuberculosis as 'the great mimic'.

The undesirable and unwanted effects of drugs are of various types. Overdosage may be absolute or relative. In 'intolerance' the characteristic effects are produced by an abnormally low drug dose. 'Idiosyncrasy' implies an uncharacteristic response. Prolonged exposure may lead to 'cumulation'. Unwanted pharmacological reactions are 'side effects'. Facultative effects depend upon the alteration of a biological balance. The teratogenic actions of certain drugs are well known. True hypersensitivity may be of any of the four classical types of allergic reaction.

Type I   Type I anaphylactic sensitivity involves IgE (reagin) in a reaction with the mast cells or basophil cells. Histamine may be liberated in some urticarial reactions.

Type II   Type II cytotoxic reactions may be due to IgG or IgM antibodies. They involve interaction between autoantibodies and antigens on the cell walls. Phagocytosis or cell death by complement activation follows and may lead to purpura.

Type III   Type III reactions are immune-complex reactions, in which the circulating antibody complexes are deposited in the tissues. Together with complement activation, this may produce vasculitis, purpura or chronic urticaria.

Type IV   Type IV reactions are delayed cell-mediated hypersensitivity reactions involving the T-lymphocytes. The reaction may cause contact dermatitis and eczema.

PATTERNS OF CUTANEOUS REACTION

Urticaria

Several mechanisms are involved in the production of urticaria. Morphine, codeine, aspirin and atropine act directly as histamine liberators from the mast cells in the dermis. Aspirin or penicillin may also cause allergic urticaria either by a Type I IgE-mediated reaction or a Type III IgG complement-fixing reaction. Rarely, more severe and complex serum sickness and anaphylactic reactions are seen. Other drugs causing urticaria are serum, toxoids, pollen vaccines, meprobamate and imipramine.

Purpura

This may be due to either drug-induced thrombocytopenia, e.g. by quinine, or to a capillaritis as a result of stimulation of antibody to a drug–capillary endothelial cell complex, as seen with the sedatives carbromal and meprobamate.

Lupus erythermatosus-like syndrome

This syndrome differs from systemic lupus erythematosus in that renal disease does not occur and rashes are less common. Drugs that can induce the lupus erythematosus-like syndrome include hydrallazine, isoniazid, penicillamine and procainamide.

Photosensitivity

Drug reactions may be phototoxic or photo-allergic. A phototoxic, non-immune, reaction occurs when photo-active drugs are present in the skin in adequate concentration and are then exposed to sufficient light of appropriate activating wavelength.

Potentially photo-toxic drugs include tetracyclines, sulphonamides, nalidixic acid and rarely griseofulvin. In the very high dosages used in renal failure, frusemide is photo-toxic.

In contrast, the photo-allergic response depends upon an immune reaction. The mechanism probably involves the alteration of the drug by light, and the attachment of the new compound to a protein, which then acts as an antigen. Chlorpromazine, chlorothiazide, sulphonamides and promethazine may all cause photo-allergic reactions.

Fixed eruptions

This is a rare but remarkable reaction in which each exposure to the offending drug produces areas of inflammation and even blistering whose borders are fixed, constant and exactly reproducible. The hands, forearms, penis and mouth are the usual sites. Tetracyclines, barbiturates, sulphonamides, phenazone, salicylates, dapsone, phenolphthalein in laxatives, oxyphenbutazone and chlordiazepoxide are the commonest causes. The mechanisms involved are not understood.

Exanthematic eruptions

This is the commonest drug reaction. It may be erythematous and macular (scarlatiniform) or maculo-papular (morbilliform) and is symmetrical. Associated fever is common. The underlying mechanism is usually allergic. Ampicillin is the commonest cause of a morbilliform reaction today, but sulphonamides, barbiturates, phenylbutazone, *para*-aminosalicylic acid and many others may be responsible. Atropine and meprobomate characteristically can cause scarlatiniform exanthemata.

Eczematous eruptions

These may be caused by sulphonamides, sulphonylureas, phenylbutazone, methyldopa, which sometimes simulates seborrhoeic dermatitis, and gold. Sometimes the primary sensitization is topical, i.e. contact dermatitis can be provoked by systemic administration of a drug, previously used topically. Examples of drugs used both topically and systemically include antibiotics, e.g. tetracyclines, fucidic acid, gentamycin; other antiseptics, e.g. iodoquinolines; and local anaesthetics of the procaine series, e.g. benzocaine, amethocaine.

Exfoliative dermatitis

This variant of eczema is one of the most dangerous drug-induced reactions and may prove fatal. Causative drugs include gold, phenylbutazone, indomethacin, allopurinol, hydantoins, sulphonylureas and *para*-aminosalicylic acid.

Pigmentation

Heavy metals such as gold and silver may form pigmented deposits in skin. Certain antimalarials such as chloroquine and mepacrine, chlorpromazine and hydantoins may cause hypermelanosis as may oral contraceptives (facial chloasma). Fixed eruptions may show pigmented relics between exacerbations. Inorganic arsenic causes 'rain-drop' pigmentation of the trunk.

Acneiform eruptions

Corticotrophin, corticosteroids, androgens in females, isoniazid, bromides and iodides may induce rashes resembling acne vulgaris.

Bullous eruptions

There are several types of bullous eruptions. The sparse large bullae seen on pressure areas after barbiturate overdosage are distinctive and are not due to immunological mechanisms. Fixed eruptions may be bullous if very intense. Sulphonamides, halides and barbiturates may induce allergic bullous reactions. Phototoxic bullae can be caused by nalidixic acid and high-dose frusemide. A pemphigus-like reaction can be caused by penicillamine.

Erythema multiforme

This hypersensitivity reaction can be caused by barbiturates, salicylates, sulphonamides (particularly the long-acting ones), penicillin, hydantoins and sulphonylureas. The same drugs rarely induce epidermal necrolysis, or scalded skin syndrome. (See p. 181.)

Lichenoid eruptions

Drug rashes mimicking lichen planus are well recognized. The mucosae and skin may both be involved. The causes include mepacrine, chloroquine, quinine, quinidine, thiazides, chlorpropamide, gold and the beta blocker, practolol, which is no longer used orally.

Psoriasiform eruptions

Methyldopa, practolol, gold and phenylbutazone may induce rashes with some features suggestive of psoriasis. Lithium salts and the antimalarials, mepacrine and chloroquine, may aggravate pre-existing psoriasis.

Drug-induced alopecia

Cytotoxic drugs, particularly cyclophosphamide, interfere with the growth or anagen phase of the hair follicle cycle. Anticoagulants and possibly oral contraceptive withdrawal can induce a premature resting, or telogen, phase, which leads to loss of hair three months later when re-growth commences. Anti-thyroid drugs may have a similar action.

Nail dystrophy

Photo-onycholysis may be one manifestation of tetracycline photo-toxicity.

Vasculitis

Blood vessel involvement is probably due to drug-induced immune complex deposition in the small vessels. The skin and kidneys are most likely to be affected. Purpuric and necrotic papules, ulceration, etc. may be seen. Sulphonamides, guanethidine, diuretics and phenytoin have been implicated.

Erythema nodosum

This is a type of vasculitis with a characteristic pattern (see p. 181). Sulphonamides, including salazopyrin, and oral contraceptives may induce this reaction.

DIAGNOSIS

Laboratory aids are almost valueless in the diagnosis of drug eruptions; analysis of the history, allied with the findings on examination is all important. All drugs taken in the three weeks prior to an acute eruption must be listed and the date of onset of therapy compared with that of the rash. Drugs introduced 7–14 days before the onset of rash are most suspect and must be arranged in rank order of suspicion on the basis of their known predilection to cause eruptions. Thus some commonly prescribed drugs virtually never cause rashes; these include digoxin, diazepam, salbutamol, frusemide in normal dosages, paracetamol, erythromycin and flucloxacillin. Ideally drugs under suspicion should be withdrawn but this must partly depend on therapeutic imperatives and whether chemically unrelated alternatives are available.

In general, discontinuation of the offending drug will lead to clearance of the rash in one to three weeks. Exceptions are penicillin urticaria, which may take months to disappear, and exfoliative dermatitis of any cause. Where several suspect drugs have been withdrawn simultaneously, readministration may be the only way of making certain of the diagnosis. This procedure is safe with fixed, lichenoid, photosensitive or acneiform eruptions but may be dangerous or even fatal with urticaria, erythema multiforme or exfoliative dermatitis. Patch testing is rarely of value and intra-dermal testing is likely to give false negative results since the offending drug is rarely a complete antigen. Patch and intra-dermal testing may also be dangerous, causing anaphylactic shock, e.g. tests with penicillin and streptomycin. There is no reliable in-vitro test although eosinophilia, basophilopenia, or low serum complement point towards a drug reaction. Skin biopsy is rarely helpful.

12

URTICARIA

Urticaria (nettle rash or hives) is a condition in which weals arise on the skin (Fig. 63). Usually the weals arise on a pink ground and itch. The lesions last half an hour to twenty four hours and then disappear without trace. Angioedema, previously called angioneurotic oedema, is a larger version of urticaria, with larger lesions and deeper swellings which may take a few days to subside. Weals are produced by vasodilatation and increased capillary permeability which allows fluid and white blood cells to pass into the dermis. The vasodilatation may be produced by histamine liberated from the mast cells in the skin but other vasoactive substances may be involved, e.g. acetylcholine, kinins and prostaglandins. 5-Hydroxytryptamine is not thought to play a significant part in urticaria.

Some urticarias are the result of immunological mechanisms. In Type I reactions IgE, produced in response to an antigen, becomes attached to the mast cells. When subsequent exposure takes place, the antigen reacts with IgE on the mast cell surfaces and histamine is produced leading to urticaria, angioedema, asthma, hay fever or anaphylactic shock. Type III reactions may produce urticaria as part of serum sickness when the antigen reacts with IgG to produce circulating complexes. Complement is involved in Type III, but not in Type I reactions. It is also involved in the rare and dangerous hereditary angioedema in which there is a deficiency of CI esterase inhibitor.

CAUSES OF URTICARIA

There are many causes of urticaria. Physical agents may be responsible. Some people are dermographic and may produce weals in response to a small scratch, rub or injury; they may then

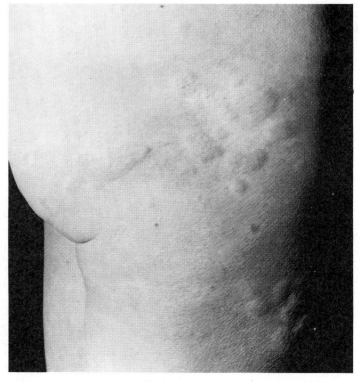

Fig. 63. Urticaria.

complain of weals and irritation without realizing that trauma is responsible. Cold, heat and light, both ultra-violet and visible, produce urticaria in some, as may food allergies. Drug allergy is an important cause. Some drugs can worsen urticaria without invoking an allergic mechanism; thus asprin and the histamine liberators, morphine and codeine, should be avoided by any patient with urticaria. Parasitic infestation may produce urticaria and dermographism. Those infected with scabies may develop secondary dermographism. Contact urticaria is unusual apart from nettle and jelly fish stings. Inhaled allergens rarely produce urticaria. Systemic diseases such as systemic lupus erythematosus, Hodgkin's disease and leukaemia may result in urticaria.

Emotional upsets and disorders are always listed as causes but one should not hurry forward with this explanation, for a patient with severe urticaria will inevitably be anxious. Emotion certainly is one of the trigger factors in cholinogenic urticaria. People with atopic eczema often develop urticaria after eating one or more food items; the food produces urticaria without any effect, good or bad, on the atopic eczema.

Cholinogenic urticaria is thought to be due to the liberation of acetylcholine from the sympathetic nerve endings of the sweat glands. The lesions are pinhead weals on large flares. Adolescents and young adults are most commonly affected. Embarrassment, heat, and exercise bring on an attack.

INVESTIGATIONS

A blood count with a high degree of eosinophilia suggests a parasitic infestation. A high ESR suggests systemic disease. Patch, intradermal and scratch tests are of surprisingly little help. In the dermographic patient, rubbing or scratching the skin with a spatula produces a brisk reaction within two minutes.

MANAGEMENT

Urticaria is usually described as either acute or chronic. Acute urticaria seldom presents a problem. It is often due to an infection, a drug or a food, and is treated symptomatically with oral antihistamines and occasionally with prednisolone. In very severe cases, intravenous antihistamine or hydrocortisone with or without subcutaneous adrenaline (epinephrine), 1:1000, 0.5 ml injected slowly, may be required.

Chronic urticaria is much more of a problem and it should be realized that it is only in a very small minority of cases that a definite cause can be found. A food diary may be useful in identifying allergens. In addition it is possible to withdraw various foods at different times. In severe cases, it may be justifiable to admit the patient to hospital on a glucose and water diet for 48 hours and then introduce foods one by one every 24 hours. Diet sheets can help in the avoidance of particular food constituents, e.g. tartrazine and other artificial food dyes, the preservative sodium benzoate, and salicylates, which are present naturally in many foods. Low nickel diets have also been devised for those sensitive to nickel. Low yeast diets may be advised but are only worth while if the candida prick test is positive (an exception to the rule that prick tests are not valuable).

It is a good idea to stop all non essential drugs that a patient may be taking in case they are the cause of the eruption. In general, stopping the offending drug produces rapid cure but there are exceptions. A penicillin injection may lead to an attack lasting for several months, presumably because of the formation and circulation of immune complexes. Aspirin, and the many medicines and tablets with other names which contain it, should be forbidden.

Antihistamines are a great and wonderful discovery and are invaluable in the treatment of urticaria. Antihistamines act by blocking the receptor sites so that histamine cannot attach itself. They are not 100% effective in controlling urticaria either because side effects limit the dose or because there are other vasoactive substances involved. It is best to familiarize oneself with a few antihistamines as there are so many. Four milligrams of chlorpheniramine (Piriton, U.K.; Chlortrimeton[R], U.S.A.), 1 mg clemastine (Tavegil) or 50 mg mebhydralin (Fabahistin, U.K.) may be given in a dose of from one to two tablets, two, three or four times a day. Promethazine (Phenergan, U.K.) or trimeprazine (Vallergan, U.K.; Temaril[R], U.S.A.) produce drowsiness in many adults and hence are best given in a single dose of 10 – 30 mg at night, since both are long acting. Patients should always be warned that antihistamine drowsiness is a side effect and they should be cautious about driving or operating machinery until they have assessed the effect on their wakefulness and reaction time. Hydroxyzine hydrochloride (Atarax, U.K.) 10 mg tablets are used especially in physical and cholinogenic urticarias. Systemic corticosteroids have a place in the treatment of severe acute urticaria, serum sickness and anaphylactic shock. Local applications are seldom necessary but Calamine lotion or a cold fluorochlorohydrocarbon (PR spray, U.K.) may be applied.

Hyposensitization is used for heat and cold urticaria. The patient takes a hot or cold bath daily which discharges the histamine in the mast cells and keeps them depleted. The treatment should be started cautiously and under antihistamine cover.

Papular urticaria is usually a reaction to insect bites.

13

PURPURA AND VASCULAR DISORDERS

PURPURA

Purpura is a symptom or a sign and there are many causes for it.
Purpura means the extravasation of blood from blood vessels into
the tissues. The lesions are blood-coloured to begin with and may
then be degraded into the colours of a fading bruise, blue-green
and yellow. A small bruise is a petechia, a large one an ecchymosis,
a raised one a haematoma. Purpura is usually subepidermal or
deeper, but in plantar warts the tiny black points which distinguish them from corns or calluses are due to altered blood in the
epidermis. Purpura does not fade on pressure which distinguishes
it from vascular erythema, telangiectasia, and all angiomata bar
one, the senile or Campbell de Morgan spot which does not blanch
on pressure. Purpura of whatever cause often appears initially on
the legs. It tends to fade fairly rapidly but may take longer on the
lower leg and indeed in those with poor venous return may remain
as haemosiderin, giving a brown discoloration (see hypostatic
dermatitis). Sometimes blood becomes trapped between the
epithelium and the submucosa on, for instance, the lip and
remains indefinitely. Raised or palpable purpura is found in
anaphylactoid purpura, in macro or cryoglobulinaemia and in vasculitis (see p. 158). Purpura may be quite trivial, e.g. a mechanical
bruise, or of the gravest importance, e.g. a severe life-threatening
infection, drug reaction or blood disease.

THROMBOCYTOPENIC PURPURA

Thrombocytopenic purpura may be idiopathic or secondary to an
infection, a drug, leukaemia, aplastic anaemia, systemic lupus
erythematosis or other autoimmune disease.

Non-Thrombocytopenic Purpura

Non-thrombocytopenic purpura may be extravascular, vascular or intravascular. Examples of the extravascular form are senile or steroid purpura where there is insufficient collagen to support the capillaries. The vascular form may be due to damage to the vessel wall by drugs, scurvy, trauma, stasis, infections, autoimmune disease, 'allergic vasculitis', the capillaritis of the dermatological purpuras, renal disease, amyloid disease or diabetes. In intravascular non-thrombocytopenic purpura the blood clots either too readily because of an excess of platelets or because a macro or cryoglobulin precipitates, or the blood does not clot sufficiently as in vitamin K deficiency, or where anticoagulants are being administered, or in disseminated intravascular coagulation.

Purpura Haemorrhagia

Purpura haemorrhagia, the idiopathic form of thrombocytopenic purpura, may present in childhood or in young adult life. It occurs in an acute and a chronic form. Epistaxis, bleeding from the gums and melaena may be features. The platelet lifespan is shortened. Treatment includes corticosteroids and blood transfusions and in the chronic type, splenectomy.

Drug-induced Purpura

Drug-induced purpura may be thrombocytopenic or non-thrombocytopenic, allergic or non-allergic. Numerous drugs are known to produce purpura: sulphonamides; gold; barbiturates; quinine and quinidine; carbromal; chlorothiazide; phenylbutazone; oxyphenbutazone; indomethacin; tetracyclines; corticosteroids; and ACTH. Some drugs such as aspirin and the anti-inflammatory rheumatoid drugs also inhibit platelet aggregation and should be avoided in haemorrhagic states. It is a good rule to stop all non essential drugs when purpura occurs. Strong local steroids produce a picture similar to senile purpura on the hands and arms, and in moist flexures.

Senile Purpura

Senile purpura occurs mainly on the extensor surface and radial border of the forearms and the backs of the hands in old people.

The lesions are dark purple bruises with irregular outlines and clear cut margins. It is due to atrophy of the dermal collagen which leaves the blood vessels unsupported so that they rupture after minor trauma.

ANAPHYLACTOID PURPURA

Anaphylactoid purpura (Henoch Schoenlein) is thought to be due to antigen-antibody damage to blood vessels but a precise cause is rarely found in a particular case. Although most common in children it may also occur in adults. The skin lesions often begin as weals which then become purpuric. The legs are the commonest site. There may be fever, malaise, colic, vomiting, joint pain and swelling, and nephritis.

SCURVY

Scurvy is seen in old people who live alone and those who for any reason do not eat a full and balanced diet. The first lesions are often purpura around the hair follicles of the thighs, later there may be ecchymoses of the saddle area (the buttocks and backs of the thighs) and woody oedema as well as ecchymoses of the lower legs. Scurvy buds of the gum occur only in those with their own teeth, particularly in the presence of gingivitis.

CAPILLARITIS

Capillaritis usually presents as purpura on the ankles and lower legs (Fig. 64). The lesions may resemble cayenne pepper or may be pigmented and lichenoid as well as purpuric. There are no blood changes as a rule. Venous insufficiency and reactions to socks, khaki uniform, rubber boots and the drug carbromal have been incriminated but in most cases the cause is obscure.

DISSEMINATED INTRAVASCULAR COAGULATION

This is a grave illness associated with Gram-negative septicaemia and other infections. Purpura which may progress to gangrene is a feature. The platelets and fibrinogen in the blood are diminished and the prothrombin time is prolonged. Heparin is used in the treatment to prevent coagulation in the vessels.

The Investigation of Purpura

A blood count, ESR and platelet count should be performed and the serum proteins estimated. If indicated the bone marrow should be examined and tests performed for cryoglobulins. Occasionally patch testing is helpful, e.g. chemicals in rubber boots may penetrate the skin and produce local purpura. A positive Hess' test is an indication of increased capillary fragility. A sphygmomanometer cuff is applied to the upper arm and inflated to just above the diastolic blood pressure. After five minutes the pressure is released. The development of more than five petechiae in a square inch (6.25 cm²) is considered abnormal.

VASCULAR DISORDERS

Damage to the large and medium sized arteries as in atheroma and arteriosclerosis may be accompanied by ischaemic pain such as intermittent claudication. Areas of gangrenous ulceration may occur affecting the extremities of the limbs. Diabetics are liable to this type of arteriopathy. Arteriosclerosis of smaller vessels produces patchy ischaemia with ulceration of the skin; the painful ulcers of the lower legs in women with hypertension are an example. Raising the limb will make the pain worse, unlike the situation in venous insufficiency. Ischaemia resulting from disease of the digital arteries may present with dystrophy of the nails, including onycholysis. The hypostatic syndromes which include hypostatic pigmentation, eczema, ulceration and atrophie blanche, are caused by venous insufficiency.

Vasculitis

Vasculitis, or more correctly angeitis, includes a wide range of disorders all characterized by inflammatory changes in the walls of medium size and small blood vessels. The clinical picture depends largely on the size and depth of the blood vessels involved ranging from polyarteritis nodosa (see p. 174) with the larger vessels, to the Henoch-Schoenlein syndrome (see p. 155) with the smallest. Vasculitis may be the result of the circulation of toxic immune complexes but it is unusual to identify the antigen which is responsible. In some syndromes the changes are necrotizing while in others they are obstructive. In those varieties involving the viscera, the prognosis can be serious but in the purely cutaneous varieties the

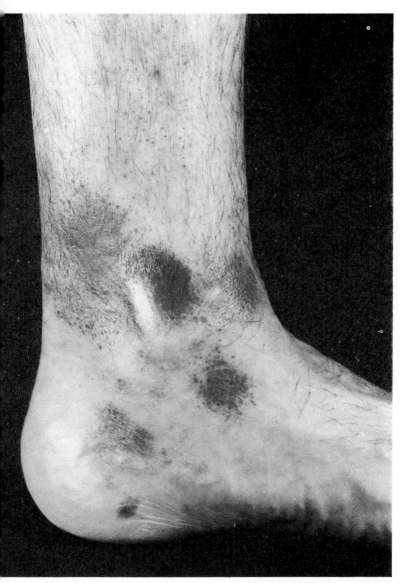

Fig. 64. Purpura due to capillaritis. Note cayenne pepper appearance.

prognosis as to life is good although relapses may continue to appear for many years. Clinical features in the skin include petechiae, red macules and papules, nodules and ulcers (Figs. 65 and 66). The commonest cutaneous variety is nodular vasculitis. It occurs chiefly on the legs of middle-aged women. The lesions, which may be tender, can be felt more easily than they can be seen. They are red, firm and deep, and are fixed to the underlying tissues. They disappear spontaneously but usually relapse repeatedly. Usually both legs are affected but the nodules are rarely symmetrical. Occasionally they ulcerate. Another syndrome has much smaller, multiple, more superficial nodules which may ulcerate, and red papules, and petechiae. Meningococcal septicaemia, erythema ncdosum (see p. 180), Bazin's disease (see p. 54) and polyarteritis nodosa form part of the differential diagnosis of nodules on the legs.

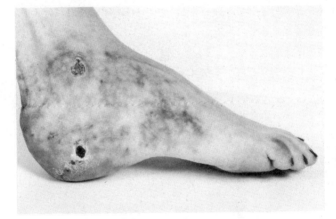

Fig. 65. Vasculitis with livedo reticularis and ulceration.

Treatment. Pain and oedema are the main problems. Antiinflammatory analgesics such as indomethacin may be of value; if not long-term prednisolone (5–10 mg daily) may be necessary. Pressure bandaging helps to control the oedema.

BUERGER'S DISEASE

Buerger's disease occurs mainly in males between 20 and 40. It is

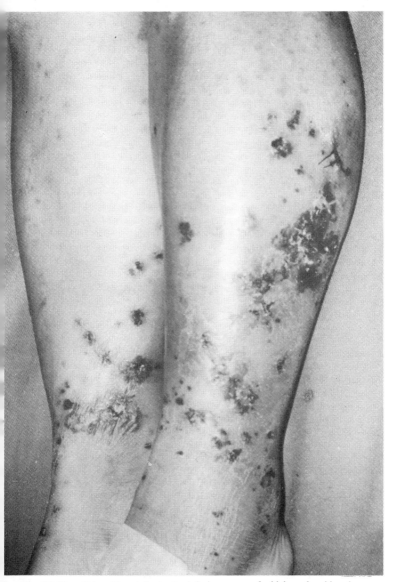

Fig. 66. Vasculitis with nodular purpuric lesions, some of which are breaking down.

rare. It affects small and medium sized arteries and superficial and deep veins. Arterial involvement produces necrosis and gangrene mainly in the legs. Venous involvement may present as thrombophlebitis migrans. It is often associated with heavy cigarette smoking, and progress of the disease, often leading to amputation, may be arrested if smoking is stopped.

VENOUS INSUFFICIENCY

Venous insufficiency is a common condition affecting the lower legs and producing pigmentation, dermatitis and ulceration. Women are much more commonly affected than men. The trouble arises because there is interference with the venous return of the blood on account of either a deep vein thrombosis or incompetence of the valves of the veins, or both. The result is venous hypertension which damages the small blood vessels of the legs. Thrombosis of the deep veins, which carry 80% of the returning blood, is the commonest cause of the trouble. It occurs after surgical operations, including cut-down drips and the injection of varicose veins, during bed rest for medical conditions, during pregnancy, as a result of taking oestrogens (e.g. the pill) or in obesity. Varicose veins are by no means an essential diagnostic indicator, because severe hypostatic ulceration can arise in their absence. Likewise, very marked varicose veins occur in some young people (probably this is hereditary), and yet their venous circulation is quite sound. Hence the terms varicose, eczema, ulcer etc. should be avoided.

Clinical picture

Oedema, pigmentation or eczema may be the first sign. Ulceration often follows trauma. The ulcers may be large or small and regular or irregular in shape. They occur in the lower third of the leg (Fig. 67), often in the region of the malleoli which may indicate that the perforator veins are incompetent (the 'ankle "blow-out" syndrome'). The leg is warm and the pulses can be felt in the absence of oedema. The ulcers are usually painless but the leg may ache, although this can be relieved by elevating the limb. These points help to distinguish hypostatic from arteriosclerotic ulcers. It may be desirable to do serological tests for syphilis. In rare instances long standing ulcers of any kind may become neoplastic and

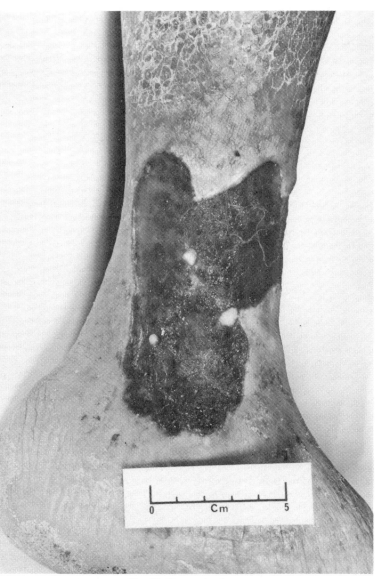

Fig. 67. Hypostatic ulcer.

biopsies should be done if there is any suspicion of this. Contact dermatitis is a frequent complication because medicaments tend to be applied for months or years. The dermatitis may appear on the affected leg but sometimes the local reaction is minimal and a widespread eczematous rash appears on the limbs and body – hence the importance of insisting on the removal of bandages from the legs when examining a patient, wherever the rash. Episodes of superficial thrombophlebitis, periphlebitis and cellulitis may lead to inflamed induration and organized oedema. Small white scars, or atrophie blanche, arising without ulceration is common in the hypostatic syndrome.

Management

Prophylaxis is better than cure! Patients should be mobilized as soon as possible after surgical operations. Exercises are mandatory for those confined to bed. Any contraceptive pill should be of the low or non-oestrogen type. Obesity should be discouraged. Those with venous insufficiency should be warned to avoid trauma to the legs. Old people should be warned against sleeping or resting all day and night in a chair.

When the only lesions present are pigmentation and purpuric puncta, no treatment is needed for the skin. Instead, as these are signs of failure in the circulatory return with the ever present threat of oedema, elastic stockings or tights should be worn. Especially valuable, although expensive, are stockings which exert a graded pressure e.g. the Jobst venous pressure gradient support. When eczematous changes have occurred, the treatment is as for eczema (see p. 142). Ambulatory treatment is used for most patients with hypostatic ulcers. If the ulcer is discharging pus or fluid, a wet dressing with equal parts of eusol and paraffin is applied and kept moist with polythene. The surrounding skin must be protected with zinc compound paste, B.P. (Lassar's paste). When the ulcer becomes dry it may be painted with magenta paint (Castellani's paint) and covered with a non-adherent dressing (Melolin, U.K.). The leg should be bandaged with an elasto-crepe or elastic web (blue line) bandage from the toes to just below the knee. If there is also eczema, it may be better to bandage the leg first with a zinc paste bandage (Viscopaste P.B. 7, U.K.; Viscopaste[R], U.S.A.), and then apply an elastic adhesive support bandage – this forms a temporary made-to-measure elastic stocking. The dressing should be changed after 3, 7 or 14 days. Too frequent changes of dressing remove the epithelium from the healing ulcers.

Patients with ulcers which resist ambulant treatment should be admitted to hospital and put to bed, with the foot of the bed raised. The leg muscles should be constantly exercised. Split skin or pinch grafts are surprisingly successful even in the most resistant cases. Diuretics may be required for the oedema. Systemic antibiotics should be given for cellulitis. A diet should be adivsed in obese persons. Anaemia should be treated. The injection of sclerosants and the surgical stripping has a part to play in the therapy of varicose veins, but neither should be undertaken unless adequate tests demonstrate that the venous return via the deep veins is satisfactory.

CHILBLAINS

Chilblains or perniosis are an exaggerated response to cold. They occur in the winter in temperate climates – usually when the temperature is just above freezing point. The fingers, the toes, the heels, the ears, and the tip of the nose are common sites, although less commonly the upper outer thighs may be affected in plump girls. Itching and burning and later pain are the symptoms. The affected areas become bright red and swollen; later cyanosis, blistering, ulceration and scarring may follow. As a rule chilblains clear when the winter weather clears, but in some there is permanent injury. Children and young people are most affected. The cause is an abnormal reaction to cold, consisting of vasospasm of the arterioles followed by vasodilatation and exudation of fluid into the tissues.

Treatment. The most effective treatment is keeping warm. A thermometer should be kept handy and the ambient temperature at home or work should be kept at 15°C (60°F) or higher if at all possible. Out of doors, warm clothing should be worn to protect the body core and the extremities. Warm gloves, stockings, trousers and footwear should be loose so as not to impede the circulation. Activity is advised for the sedentary and lethargic. Vasodilators such as nicotinic acid 100 mg or thymoxamine 40 mg three or four times a day may be prescribed. If the skin is broken, 0.25% chlortetracycline ointment may be applied. An ointment containing phenol 1%, camphor 4%, Balsam of Peru 2% in equal parts of lanolin and soft paraffin is comforting for intact skin.

RAYNAUD'S PHENOMENON

Commoner in females than males, Raynaud's phenomenon affects the hands and sometimes the feet. Exposure to even moderate cold induces arteriolar spasm producing first of all pallor then reactive erythema or cyanosis. It may be an isolated symptom but may also occur in systemic sclerosis or systemic lupus erythematosus. The use of vibrating tools such as a pneumatic drill may also produce the phenomenon.

BED SORES

Bed sores (pressure sores, decubitus ulcers) arise as a consequence of interference with the capillary blood flow by prolonged pressure. They occur mainly in those confined to bed by debilitating disease or diseases which impair movement e.g. arthritis and neurological disease. The commonest sites are the sacral area, over the trochanters, the malleoli and the heels. The first sign is erythema, later superficial ulceration occurs followed sometimes by deep ulceration, even down to the bone. Maceration of the skin may be a contributing factor and secondary infection is a complication. Prevention is more successful than cure. The invalid who cannot move himself should be turned every two hours, if necessary using a turning frame. Ripple beds, water beds, applying plastic or rubber foam to bony points and nursing the patient on a sheepskin are also helpful. The skin should be kept clean and dry. Ulcers should be treated with magenta paint (Castellani's paint), eusol and paraffin in equal parts, chlortetracycline or gentamycin ointment. A high protein diet or the correction of anaemia may also be necessary.

NEUROPATHIC ULCERS

Neuropathic ulcers may be mentioned in relation to the above because they are also the result of inappropriate pressure to the skin. These ulcers arise because sensation is impaired and the warning signals of injury fail to alert the patient. Diabetic neuropathy is the commonest cause of neuropathic ulceration but leprosy, lumbo-sacral nerve compression, syringomyelia and, classically, tabes dorsalis may be responsible.

14

AUTOIMMUNE DISEASES

The autoimmune diseases are thought nowadays to be the result of a disturbance in the immune mechanism possibly induced by a virus so that the body produces antibodies against its own constituents. The evidence for this is not conclusive but includes the production of similar diseases in animals by immunological manipulation and the demonstration of abnormalities in humans by immunofluorescent studies. Pemphigus and pemphigoid, which may well be autoimmune disorders, are dealt with for convenience in the chapter on bullous eruptions. Vitiligo and alopecia areata are also discussed elsewhere.

LUPUS ERYTHEMATOSUS

There are two principal forms of this malady: chronic discoid lupus erythematosus (discoid LE) and systemic lupus erythematosus (SLE). The commoner form, discoid LE, is an intractable chronic eruption affecting the exposed parts in both sexes, partucularly the nose and the adjacent areas of the cheeks; the lesions are erythematous and discoid, with a tendency to form thin scales, and are associated with follicular plugging. The eruption characteristically results in scarring without ulceration. The other principal form, SLE, is rare and is so different in its manifestations that some consider that it should not be regarded as an acute form of the same disease. It is usually a malady of women of child-bearing age and is associated with signs and symptoms which often include debility, arthralgia, neuro-psychiatric disorders, albuminuria, leucopenia, toxaemia, endocarditis, polyserositis, and sometimes a generalized eruption and loss of hair.

Aetiology

Lupus erythematosus is more common in women than in men. The ratio of incidences, male:female, is 1:2 for discoid LE and 1:8 for SLE. It seldom develops before the age of 17 years or after the age of 48 years; the highest incidence is amongst persons between 30 and 35 years of age. Genetic factors are thought to be important, resulting in 'forbidden clones' of lymphocytes which produce cellular auto-antibodies. Sensitivity to light determines the fact that the site of election of the rash is the face and exposed parts; acute exacerbations of sub-acute or chronic lupus erythematosus may arise as a result of injudicious exposure to the sun or ultraviolet rays. Drugs such as sulphonamides, hydrallazine, penicillamine and many others may induce an SLE syndrome. Some drugs produce an exacerbation of existing SLE and discoid LE, particularly sulphonamides, penicillin, streptomycin and hydantoin.

Pathology

The capillaries of the dermis are dilated and in the systemic form the vessels may show fibrinoid degeneration. There is a marked infiltration with small round cells, which is associated with oedema. The collagen and elastic fibres undergo degeneration. The horny layer of the epidermis is thickened, but the outer layers of the epidermis are markedly diminished in size. It is characteristic of the chronic type of the disease that the pilosebaceous orifices are plugged with horny cells. There is liquefaction of the basal cell layer. Immunofluorescence reveals deposition of IgG, IgM and complement at the dermoepidermal junction of the affected skin. in SLE IgG may be found in sun-exposed normal skin and immune complexes and complement may be deposited in the kidneys.

Chronic discoid lupus erythematosus

This disease commences as a fixed erythema. Later scaling telangiectasia and scarring develop. If the scale is lifted, carpet tack prolongations into pilosebaceous orifices, which are the result of the formation of horny plugs, can be seen. The scaling is seldom seen in its full glory nowadays because most patients are using local steroid preparations. The lesions spread peripherally, and are covered with thin adherent scales. After persisting for a variable time (usually months or years), healing occurs in the centre of each area and a white tissue-paper scar is formed. The lesions usually appear in small groups or discs, and the sites of election are the cheeks and nose, although the forehead, scalp, ears, the 'V' of the neck and hands may be affected (Plate IX). The eruption tends to be symmetrical, and the classical appearance of 'bat's-wing lupus' is caused by discoid lesions breaking out on each cheek and spreading over the nose. In coloured people both hyperpigmentation and hypopigmentation may be seen in the lesions. The disease is not preceded or accompanied by malaise, and the eruption itself is painless.

Systemic lupus erythematosus

Systemic lupus erythematosus affects many organs of the body. The skin signs, which may be entirely absent, are:

1. The discoid LE picture, especially in those who start with discoid and progress to SLE.

2. Bright red erythema of the face including the butterfly area and other uncovered parts is often related to exposure to the sun.

3. Erythema and erosions of the mouth and lips.

4. Erythema of the palms and peringual erythema.

5. Splinter haemorrhages and small infarcts of the finger tips.

6. Urticaria.

7. Diffuse alopecia especially affecting the sides of the scalp.

The involvement of other systems may produce fever, arthralgia, pleurisy, pneumonitis, pericarditis and Libman-Sacks endocarditis, proteinuria, mental and neurological disturbance, nausea, vomiting, abdominal pain, ocular haemorrhage and retinal cytoid bodies.

Diagnosis and prognosis

Diagnosis of the chronic discoid form of the disease is not difficult unless the patient has had treatment before coming under observation. There are no 'apple-jelly' nodules, as in lupus vulgaris; the scales are more delicate and smaller than those of psoriasis, and are more firmly attached to the skin than those formed in seborrhoeic conditions. They also show the characteristic horny plugs described above. A biopsy of the affected skin is very helpful.

The diagnosis of SLE is often difficult in the early stages, but assistance can often be obtained by demonstrating antinuclear factors e.g. anti-DNA antibody, or LE cells in the laboratory. Raised ESR, hypergammaglobulinaemia, anaemia and leucopenia are often features. Low serum complement may herald active phases of SLE.

Discoid lupus erythematosus runs a long course with remissions and exacerbations, although scarring has been much less of a danger with the use of the new powerful local steroids. SLE, once regarded as a death sentence, is still a dangerous disease, but has a better prognosis than was previously thought, partly because milder cases of SLE are diagnosed with increasing frequency and partly because systemic steroids have probably reduced the mortality. In one large series there was a 50% survival rate after ten years.

Treatment

Discoid LE is best treated with very strong, strong or medium strength local steroid ointments or creams. Intralesional triamcinolone acetonide injections or flurandrenalone tape (Haelan, U.K.; Cordran[R], U.S.A.) may also be used. Chloroquine administered by mouth in small doses has a considerable suppressive effect. However, it may rarely produce blindness as the result of damage to the retina, and hence expert supervision is required. The patient should avoid sunlight and intense cold. The prescription of 'sunscreens' should be considered. Expert advice for cosmetic camouflage should be sought in appropriate instances. SLE requires systemic steroids during exacerbations. Renal involvement is regarded as especially dangerous and azothioprine, cyclophosphamide or methotrexate are often required as well as the systemic steroids.

DERMATOMYOSITIS

Dermatomyositis is a disease with a characteristic rash associated with muscular weakness. Commonly it occurs in children under ten years or adults between 40 and 60. The cause is not known but it is regarded as an autoimmune disorder. In the adult group there is an associated internal carcinoma or reticulosis in about a third of patients. The pathology of the skin is similar to that of lupus erythematosus; the affected muscles show degeneration of the muscle fibres and an increase in the number of sarcolemmal nuclei. The onset may be acute with fever, or insidious. There is swelling of the skin, heliotrope erythema of the eyelids and upper face, and a fixed erythema with atrophy and telangiectasia over the bony points, the knees, the elbows and in a linear distribution over the dorsal surfaces of the fingers and hands. Weakness with or without pain and tenderness of the proximal muscles of the limbs and perhaps of the muscles of swallowing, speaking and breathing may develop. Calcification may occur in the affected limbs. The muscular weakness may exist without the skin changes (polymyositis) and vice versa.

Diagnosis and treatment

Increase in urinary creatine and raised levels of the enzymes concerned with muscle breakdown in the serum, i.e. aldolase, creatine phosphokinase, lactic dehydrogenase and transaminases, are often found. The electromyograph is abnormal and biopsy of an affected muscle is helpful. Antinuclear factor is usually absent. In the early stages, poliomyelitis and trichinosis must be distinguished. In some cases it may be difficult to distinguish from systemic sclerosis and SLE. Allergic contact dermatitis produces swelling of the eyelids also, but here irritation is a marked feature and there is no myopathy. The adult cases which have an associated neoplasm have a bad prognosis. Cases with calcinosis carry a good prognosis as regards life, but are liable to develop contractures and deformities.

Systemic steroids in high dosage are required in most cases with acute onset and in other cases with exacerbations. Immunosuppressive drugs, such as azothioprine, methotrexate, and cyclophosphamide may be required in severe cases. Physiotherapy and measures to prevent deformity are needed in chronic cases.

MORPHOEA

Morphoea is a type of scleroderma, which means hard skin. It is commoner in the female. The epidermis is often atrophic and the dermal appendages and subcutaneous fat are diminished. The dermal collagen becomes oedematous and then thickened. Morphoea is a benign though often disfiguring malady. Well defined, flat plaques of various sizes, usually round or oval in shape, develop; the adjacent skin may have a pink or violet hue. The affected skin is white, smooth and hard. Loss of hair at the sites of involvement, ulceration, or firm attachment of a plaque to underlying bone may occur. After a long period the lesions become softer and may assume a brown hue.

The vesicles tend to form in small clusters and may enlarge to form bullae. In some instances the vesicles form circular patterns and may coalesce. The lesions become modified by scratching and by secondary infections. Scars are formed only when the lesions have been deeply excoriated or have become infected. In a small percentage of cases the buccal mucous membrane is involved, but never severely. Lesions may also occur on the genital mucosa and rarely on the pharynx, larynx, and oesophagus.

The disease must be distinguished from scabies and nocturnal irritation and the distribution may help here. In dermatitis herpetifomis the lesions have usually been decapitated as soon as they appeared, because this relieves the irritation. If there is an intact lesion, biopsy is most helpful. In many cases where there is no lesion suitable for biopsy a small piece of normal skin can be submitted for immunofluorescence. Deposits of IgA in the papillae or just below the epidermis are characteristic. Failing this, a therapeutic test with dapsone or sulphapyridine may be made.

Complete remissions occur only in small minority of cases.

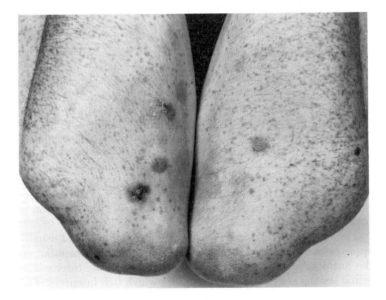

Fig. 69. Dermatitis herpetiformis. The elbows are a characteristic site.

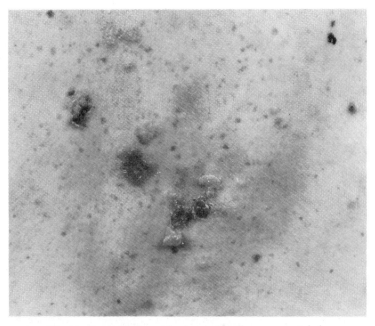

Fig. 70. Dermatitis herpetiformis: small bullae, some scratched.

Usually, however, the eruption is most severe at the onset, slowly decreases in severity, but rarely disappears permanently. Some suffer severely from the malady; in others the eruption may only be moderate or mild.

Treatment. Dapsone suppresses the lesions in the majority of patients. It must be continued as long as the disease persists and in the smallest dose which is effective. It is given as dapsone tablets B.P.C.; 100 mg a day as a starting dose is sufficient in most patients. The maximum dose is 300 mg daily. Dapsone may produce haemolytic anaemia. Cyanosis also occurs as the result of methaemoglobin formation. Sulphapyridine 1 to 3 g daily is an alternative. A strict gluten-free diet will also control the disease, or at any rate diminish the dapsone requirement. The benefits of the diet do not become apparent for several months or years. Medicines containing iodine should be avoided because they make dermatitis herpetiformis worse.

Herpes Gestationis

Herpes gestationis is similar to dermatitis herpetiformis or pemphigoid but it occurs during pregnancy and clears after the birth of the child. It may also recur with oral contraceptive therapy which should be avoided. The cause is not clear. Systemic prednisolone may be needed.

Pemphigoid

This is an uncommon disease occurring in elderly people, but nevertheless it is more common than true pemphigus. It begins with tense, occasionally haemorrhagic, bullae on the limbs or trunk in a centrifugal pattern, sometimes on an erythematous or urticarial base (Fig. 71). The mucous membranes are rarely

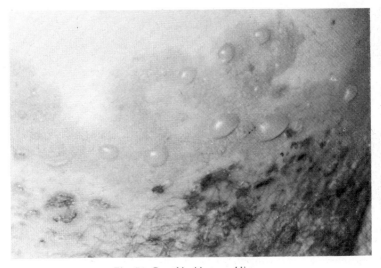

Fig. 71. Pemphigoid: tense blisters.

affected. Histologically there is a dermoepidermal blister, and no acantholysis. Immunofluorescence demonstrates IgG antibody at the dermoepidermal junction.

The course of the disease is variable. It may be steadily progressive or there may be spontaneous remissions. Although the disease is not in itself usually fatal, old people suffering from it may die in a very few years from some intercurrent malady. It can generally be controlled by treatment with corticosteroids though a maintenance dose may have to be taken for some time.

Pemphigus Vulgaris

Pemphigus vulgaris is a disease in which bullae appear in crops on apparently normal skin and mucous membrane; at the outset the constitutional symptoms are comparatively slight, but, untreated, the malady may be fatal. Persons of all ages and of both sexes may be affected, but the disease usually occurs in the 'middle years' of life. Although the cause is unknown the high incidence among persons of the Jewish ancestry suggests a genetic factor. A pemphigus-like syndrome has been reported in patients being treated with penicillamine, phenylbutazone, irgapyrin and rifampicin. There is an endemic form of the disease in Brazil called fogo selvagem.

The bullae develop in the prickle cell layer of the epidermis, where, at the outset, the intercellular fibrils disappear. The free cells soon die, their cytoplasm becomes homogeneous and their nuclei fragmented. This process, known as acantholysis, precedes the formation of bullae which are formed by cleavage in the damaged rete by fluid which probably is derived from the vessels of the corium. Acantholysis is a diagnostic feature in pemphigus vulgaris.

Direct and indirect immunoflorescence demonstrate that there is antibody deposition in the intercellular area between the prickle cells. This can be used as a useful diagnostic test and also suggests that pemphigus may be an autoimmune disease.

Signs and Symptoms. The eruption begins with blisters in the mouth in 35% to 40% of cases and later, similar lesions appear on the trunk or limbs. The face and scalp may also be affected. The distribution is more centripetal than in pemphigoid. The bullae usually erupt in crops, but may occur singly. They vary considerably in size and shape, and may be small or as large as a tangerine orange. The surrounding skin is normal in all respects. The bullae are flaccid and rupture easily (unlike those of pemphigoid). The raw surfaces left tend to extend themselves and have little tendency to spontaneous healing. Constitutional symptoms are slight. The temperature may rise when the bullae erupt, but rapidly returns to normal. Pemphigus was fatal in 80% of cases within five years before effective treatment became available. With modern therapy two thirds or more survive 10 years and many 20 years. Nowadays death is more likely to be due to the complications of therapy than to the disease itself. Biopsy and immunofluorescence tests confirm the diagnosis.

Treatment. Prednisone is given in a dosage between 180 and 240 mg a day until the disease is controlled. The dose is then reduced quite rapidly to a maintenance level. Azothioprine, methotrexate or cyclophosphamide may be introduced to lessen the dose of the steroid. The blisters should be pricked and counted each day as a measure of the effectiveness of therapy. A non-adherent dressing should be applied to the raw surfaces. Antibiotics, either systemic or local, may be needed if there is infection. A proportion of patients will be able to stop therapy after several months or years, the rest require life-long treatment.

16

ERYTHEMA MULTIFORME AND ERYTHEMA NODOSUM

ERYTHEMA MULTIFORME

Erythema multiforme is an acute and sometimes recurrent erythema with target, or iris, lesions with or without bullae. Herpes simplex is a common precipitant and recurrence of the herpes may lead to recurrent erythema multiforme. Other viral infections such as vaccination and bacterial and mycoplasma pneumoniae infections may also induce attacks. Drugs are an important cause, especially barbiturates and sulphonamides, and particularly the long acting ones. Other associations include lupus erythematosus, leukaemia and deep radiotherapy for malignant disease. Histology shows dilation of the blood vessels of the skin and a cellular infiltrate round the vessels. The bullae are subepidermal and the overlying epidermis shows oedema or necrosis. Clinically the lesions are usually symmetrically disposed on the flexor aspects of the forearms, on the hands and elsewhere. They are red and round and become oedematous like urticaria. They often progress to form target or erythema iris lesions, which are a series of concentric rings of erythema or cyanosis, perhaps with a blister at the centre or as one of the rings. Other lesions are bullae arising on a red background. The lesions scale, crust or form erosions which heal. An attack lasts from two to six weeks but some are liable to recurrent attacks. The Stevens-Johnson syndrome is a severe febrile form of erythema multiforme in which erosive stomatitis and haemorrhagic cheilitis occur. The eyes are inflamed and there are often erosions in the anal and genital regions. The skin lesions are those described above. Bullous erythema multiforme may be confused with pemphigus, but in the latter disease there is no erythema.

Treatment. Non-vital drugs should be stopped in case they are causal. Soothing local applications should be applied, e.g.

calamine lotion or 0.25% oxytetracycline ointment. In severe cases, prednisone, 60 mg daily initially, should be given, with an antibiotic to cover if necessary. If a drug is responsible, the patient should be warned and it should be recorded in the notes, for a second attack could be fatal.

Erythema Nodosum

Erythema nodosum is most common in childhood and young adult life with females out-numbering males. It usually begins with malaise, fever and pain in the joints and limbs. Later, bright red painful and tender nodules appear, usually on the shins. The nodules may measure between 1 and 8 cm in diameter and there may be substantial oedema. A particular lesion fades in two to three weeks often showing the coloration of a bruise in the process (Plate XI). It is not uncommon to have a series of nodules over the course of six to eight weeks. Erythema nodosum is a reaction to a variety of agents, e.g. sarcoidosis, primary tuberculosis, a streptococcal sore throat, and drugs such as sulphonamide or the pill. Other causes include vaccination, Yersinia infections, North American blastomycosis, coccidomycosis, ulcerative colitis and Crohn's disease. The differential diagnosis includes nodular vasculitis (see p. 160) and Bazin's disease (see p. 54) which both have a more prolonged course. 'Erythema nodosum leprosum' is an exanthem associated usually with the treatment of leprosy; it is more widespread and pleomorphic than erythema nodosum. Chronic meningococcal septicaemia may produce smaller nodules on the legs and elsewhere.

A chest X-ray, blood count, ESR, tuberculin test (beginning with 1:10 000) and a throat swab should be done, as well as any additional tests suggested by the history and by local experience.

Treatment. If the patient is febrile and in pain, rest in bed and analgesics are recommended. In milder cases elastic bandages to the legs are helpful. Naturally, attention should be paid to the precipitating cause, e.g. causative drugs should be stopped and tuberculosis treated.

17

GRANULOMAS OF UNKNOWN ORIGIN

SARCOIDOSIS

Sarcoidosis is a disease in which epithelioid cell granulomas develop and produce multisystem disease in the chest, skin, eye, lymph glands, spleen, nervous system etc. The cause is unknown. T-cell function is depressed and B-cell activity is increased.

The skin is involved in 25% of the cases. Erythema nodosum with hilar lymphadenopathy may be the presenting symptom and this type of sarcoidosis carries a good prognosis (see p. 182). Other lesions are papules, plaques and subcutaneous swellings. Swelling and infiltration of the skin of the nose is a feature of one type, lupus pernio. In blacks, in whom sarcoidosis is common, hypopigmentation over the infiltrations may be seen, and should be differentiated from leprosy. Scars may light up and become livid when sarcoidosis develops. The usual age of onset is between 20 and 40 years. Essentially the skin lesions are non-ulcerating, non-caseating granulomas. A biopsy of a lesion or of an inflamed scar is usually characteristic. The Kveim-Silzbach test is positive in 75% of cases and the tuberculin reaction negative in 60%. The immunoglobulins and serum calcium are often raised. The chest should always be X-rayed for hilar adenopathy or parenchymal lung involvement. The differential diagnosis is from other granulomas, tuberculosis, leprosy, syphilis, cutaneous leishmaniasis, deep mycoses and beryllium, zirconium and silica granulomas.

There is no ideal treatment. For skin lesions a medium, strong or very strong corticosteroid ointment or cream should be used, or corticosteroid may be injected into indurated lesions. When the patient is generally ill or when renal function is threatened, systemic corticosteroids are advised. Chloroquine by mouth has also been used.

GRANULOMA ANNULARE

Granuloma annulare is a common condition in which there is granulomatous infiltrate in the corium, surrounding foci of collagen degeneration. The cause is obscure. One modern view is that an antigen-antibody reaction is responsible. Commonest in children and young adults, granuloma annulare can occur at any age. There is a disseminated adult type which may be associated with diabetes but no such association is found in the more common localized childhood type. The most frequent sites are the extensor aspect of the hands, arms, feet and legs. The lesions are papules or

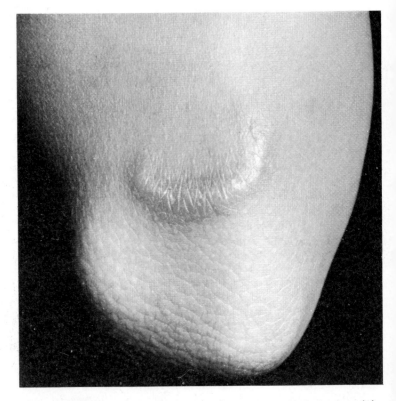

Fig. 72. Granuloma annulare. Unlike ringworm, the lesion is in the dermis, and the epidermis normal.

nodules which are skin-coloured, red or red-blue. The lesions often form a ring or a part of a ring (Fig. 72). The diagnosis from ringworm is not difficult because granuloma annulare is sited in the dermis and the epidermis is normal, whereas ringworm produces epidermal changes, scaling, vesiculation or pustulation. Granuloma annulare and rheumatoid nodules are histologically similar but the latter are usually deeper. The condition has a strong tendency to get better spontaneously, and most patients who have been assured that it has no sinister implications are happy without active treatment. Granuloma annulare can be influenced by local corticosteroids, either ointments or creams, or by intra-lesion injections.

NECROBIOSIS LIPOIDICA DIABETICORUM

This is a rare disease, which is commoner in women and tends to affect the shins, although other areas may be involved. It begins as a red plaque, later the centre becomes atrophic and translucent so that the blood vessels may be seen through the skin, while the edges become yellow or brown or remain red. The histology has similarities to granuloma annulare. Although there is a significant association with diabetes, the condition can occur in non-diabetics.

18

PSORIASIS

Psoriasis is a very common, chronic, non-infective, inflammatory skin disease characterized by the presence of sharply defined salmon-red plaques with a scaly surface.

Psoriasis is found in about 2% of the population in N.W. Europe and N. America, and is probably less common in the yellow-brown and black races. The sex ratio is probably equal. Although psoriasis can start in infancy, onset before four years is rare and before eight years uncommon. The peaks of incidence are seen in the second and third decades but the disease may begin at any age, even in senility.

Aetiology and Pathogenesis

The predisposition to psoriasis is inherited multifactorially. This has been established by population surveys, twin studies and family pedigree analyses. Strong positive correlations of psoriasis with the leucocyte histocompatibility antigen HLA – CW6 have been demonstrated, as have associations with certain blood group antigens. Carrying combinations of these genetic markers increases the risk of developing the disease, but there are ethnic variations and psoriasis can develop in the absence of these antigens. It thus seems that psoriasis is a polygenic disease, the predisposition depending on the presence of a number of genes, whose combined action draws the patient closer to a threshold beyond which environmental factors can precipitate clinical disease.

The provocative factors include trauma, for instance a cat scratch or operational incision; infection, particularly the role of streptococcal pharyngitis in precipitating guttate psoriasis of childhood; and hormonal disturbance, especially childbirth. Less common precipitating factors are sunlight, although it improves the condition in the majority, drugs such as chloroquine and lithium, hypocalcaemia and psychological stress.

Exciting strides in understanding the pathogenesis of psoriasis have taken place in the last 15 years, the landmarks being the recognition that both the epidermis and dermis are involved and that clinically unaffected skin is abnormal. The active, psoriatic epidermis is hyperkinetic with increased mitoses and an expanded basal germinative cell population. Production of new cells is increased by a factor of 20 to 30 leading to an increased epidermal volume, i.e. acanthosis. Epidermal turn-over or replacement time is shortened from the normal 30–45 days to as little as seven days. The rate of nail growth is also increased.

At present it is controversial whether the epidermal maturation defect, which results in the abnormal scaly stratum corneum, is the result of accelerated epidermopoiesis or whether the latter is compensatory and due to a feed-back mechanism, i.e. secondary to a maturation fault. It is possible that both epidermal abnormalities are due to autoimmune reactions since cell-bound antibody is formed to epidermal basal nuclei. In addition, quite separate autoimmune reactions involving a stratum corneum antigen result in the formation of immune complexes which are strongly leucotactic. This results in the migration of polymorphonuclear leucocytes into the epidermis to form the Munro micro-abscesses which are so characteristic histologically.

The epidermal changes can be summarized as acanthosis with striking epidermo-dermal infolding, parakeratosis, i.e. the formation of an abnormal nucleated loose scaly stratum corneum, absence of the stratum granulosum and the presence of polymorph micro-abscesses. The equally important dermal changes are capillary hypertrophy in the papillae and a superficial infiltrate of mainly lymphocytes and macrophages.

THE CLINICAL PICTURE

The expression of psoriasis is enormously varied, both in space and time. The disease may be trivial or universal, transient or chronic over decades with every variation between these extremes. The clinical spectrum is complicated by morphological variants and curious locations but most adult psoriasis is characteristic and easily recognizable. It is known as discoid psoriasis (Fig. 73). The

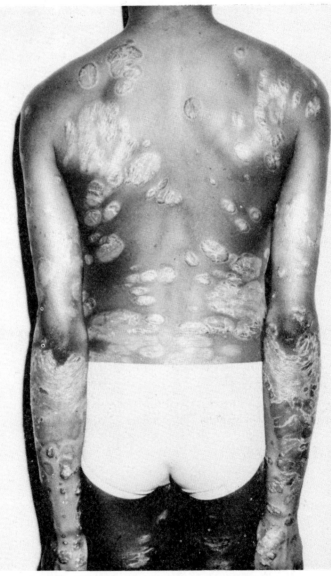

Fig. 73. Discoid psoriasis in a black patient.

plaque is sharply defined and is palpable. The colour is red with a dull salmon-coloured hue. It is covered by a white scale which is easily detached by scraping, and bleeding points are easily provoked. The scratched scale assumes a silvery colour (Fig. 74). The

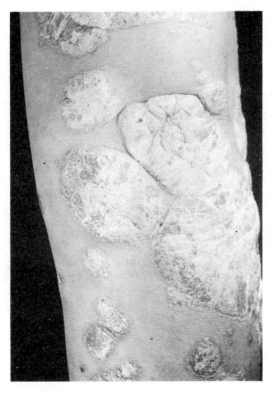

Fig. 74. Discoid psoriasis. Note silvery scale.

primary papule can grow into a plaque of any size or may coalesce to form 'geographic' patterns. Discoid psoriasis has a predilection for the extensor aspects of the limbs, especially the points of the elbows or knees, the lower back and the scalp, especially at its margins.

There are many variants of this classical picture.

Napkin psoriasis

Eruptions spreading from the napkin area in infants may be sharply defined and psoriasiform. The occurrence of this rash in babies of psoriatic families and the occasional later emergence of typical psoriasis support the belief that it occurs in infants with the psoriatic diathesis. (Fig. 75.)

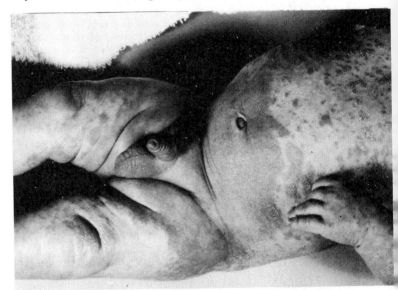

Fig. 75. Napkin psoriasis.

Guttate psoriasis

Guttate psoriasis is an acute exanthematic papular psoriasis, uniformly distributed on the trunk and limbs and often precipitated by an upper respiratory infection. It is usually seen in children but can occur in adults. (Fig 76.)

Flexural psoriasis

In some patients, particularly the elderly, psoriasis affects the axillary, sub-mammary and ano-genital folds (Fig. 77). The scale is rubbed off by intertriginous friction leaving smooth, glazed but well defined plaques.

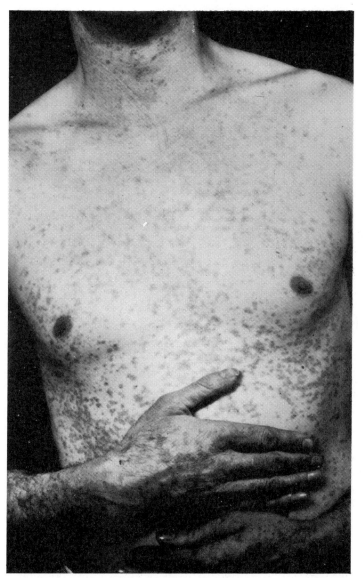

Fig. 76. Guttate psoriasis.

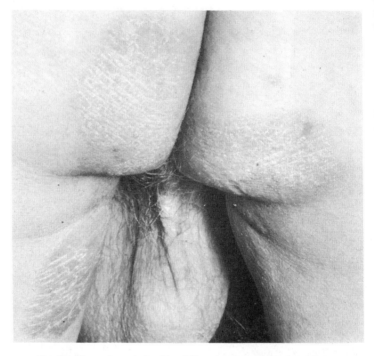

Fig. 77. Flexural psoriasis. The differential diagnosis is from tinea.

Pustular psoriasis

Uncommonly the epidermal micro-abscesses become exaggerated and macroscopic so that visible yellow pustules are set in the psoriatic skin. Such pustules are sterile. This pattern is seen usually in middle life as an indolent eruption of the palms or soles where the pustules slowly desiccate to leave discrete brown stains in the desquamating stratum corneum. The thenar and hypothenar eminences, heels and insteps are particularly affected. Rarely, pustular psoriasis may be generalized, acute and even fulminant (see Complications).

Rupioid psoriasis

This is a variant of pustular psoriasis in which heaped up, conical, orange-yellow papules form. It is indistinguishable from the 'keratoderma blenorrhagica' described in some cases of Reiter's syndrome.

Localized patterns

Some of the variants described above have characteristic locations but ordinary discoid psoriasis may also be peculiarly localized. It will not escape recognition if simple rules of diagnosis are remembered. Thus, psoriasis confined to the scalp may be misdiagnosed as dandruff. The important features are the patchy, particularly marginal, involvement and the fact that lesions are palpable as well as visible. Pruritus ani or vulvae may be due to solitary psoriatic plaques. Persistent lesions on the glans penis are not uncommon.

Psoriasis of the nails

Psoriasis affects the nails at some time in up to 50% of patients. It may disturb the matrix or the nail bed (hyponychium). Matrix disease causes pitting (Fig. 78) or ridging of the emerging nail plate (Fig. 79). Nail bed psoriasis leads to separation of the plate (onycholysis), particularly at the free end laterally (Fig. 80), and sub-ungual heaped up parakeratosis. The latter is particularly

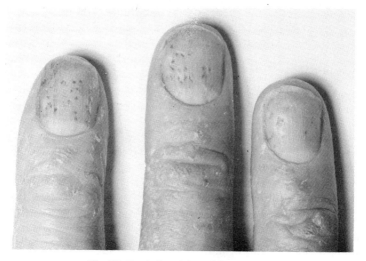

Fig. 78. Psoriasis: pitting of finger nails.

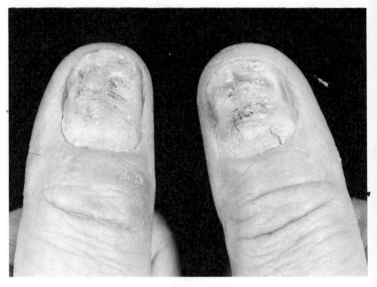

Fig. 79. Psoriasis: horizontal ridging of nails.

common in the toes whereas pitting is seen more in the finger nails.

Onycholysis may be complicated by sub-ungual bacterial colon-ization leading to a greenish-black discoloration. Rarely gross involvement of the terminal fingers leads to complete disorganiza-tion of nails with heaped up psoriasis of the nail bed and peri-onychial skin. Such acral psoriasis is particularly seen in associa-tion with arthritis and Reiter's syndrome.

COMPLICATIONS

Complications of psoriasis include erythroderma, generalized pustulation and their metabolic sequelae and polyarthritis.

In erythrodermic, or generalized exfoliative, psoriasis, the local-ized plaques are submerged in a universal inflammation of the skin. Involvement of nails, palms and soles is gross and much hair may be lost. The skin is bright red, oedematous and uncomfort-able. Exfoliation of scales may be profuse and continuous. This pattern is rare, occurs in adults and may run a sub-acute or chronic course. It occurs spontaneously but can be precipitated by injudicious topical therapy, drug reactions and cortico-steroid withdrawal.

In acute generalized pustular psoriasis, fever, nausea and toxicity usher in a fierce skin inflammation which may rapidly become universal. Masses of pin-head pustules erupt, coalesce and desquamate in crops. A leucocytosis is usual. Attacks may be fatal but fortunately this complication is rare.

Both of these forms of psoriasis may cause serious constitutional disturbance. Thermo-regulation is disturbed, cutaneous vasodilatation causing excessive heat loss with the danger of hypothermia in a cold environment. Conversely, in high ambient temperatures, hyperthermia is possible because the psoriatic skin is anhidrotic, due to blockage of the sweat ducts in the disordered epidermis. Cutaneous blood flow is greatly increased, demanding an increased cardiac output. If the cardio-vascular system is compromised by disease, cardiac embarrassment and then failure may supervene. Persistent exfoliation represents a protein loss since keratin is a fibrous protein. Hypo-albuminaemia may ensue. Transepidermal insensible water loss is also greatly increased due

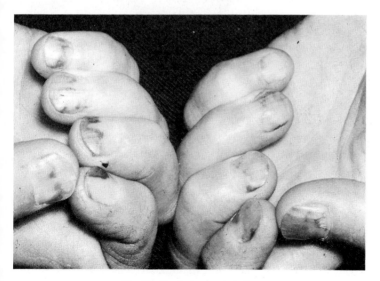

Fig. 80. Psoriasis: onycholysis.

to the impaired barrier qualities of psoriatic skin but cutaneous electrolyte loss is not a problem. Other secondary metabolic problems may include malabsorption, hypocalcaemia and folate deficiency which is partly due to increased utilization.

Psoriatic arthritis

Psoriasis and an inflammatory polyarthritis are seen together more often than chance alone would dictate. The arthritis is similar to rheumatoid but, in its classical form, has a predilection for the distal inter-phalangeal joints of the fingers and the small joints of the toes. In the fingers, the distal joint is swollen and tender (Fig. 81) and may be fixed in flexion. The adjacent nail is likely to show

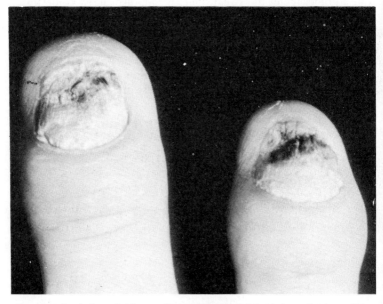

Fig. 81. Psoriatic arthritis: swelling of terminal interphalangeal joints. Note psoriasis of adjacent nail.

psoriatic changes. Sausage-like deformity of the toes is characteristic but the lateral deviation of rheumatoid is absent because the metacarpo–phalangeal and metatarso–phalangeal joints are relatively spared. Rheumatoid sub-cutaneous nodules are absent. Radiographs reveal an erosive arthropathy. Rarely, in psoriatic arthritis mutilans, joint destruction and bone lysis may be extreme and can be followed by bony ankylosis, functionally destroying the hands. However, many patients have an arthritis very similar to rheumatoid, but tending to be less symmetrical and with more spinal involvement. The only important differentiating laboratory feature in all of these groups is the absence of serum rheumatoid factors so that the Rose-Waaler and latex fixation tests give negative results.

MANAGEMENT

Psoriasis is a chronic relapsing disease for which the physician can offer suppression but not cure. The patient therefore needs social and psychological support as well as physical remedies. Attention should always be paid to any accompanying disease, such as arthritis, anaemia or depression, which may critically lower the patient's tolerance of his disability. Its non-infective nature should be stressed. Most psoriasis is treated topically; systemic therapy, which is more hazardous, is reserved for severe and disabling disease.

Topical therapy

Tar, dithranol and corticosteroids are of accepted value. Detergent shampoos, salicylic acid ointments and pastes and short wave ultra-violet light (UVB) are adjuncts to treatment.

Coal and wood tar extracts are often effective, probably by virtue of their weak anti-mitotic action. Coal tar solution B.P.C. (100 ml to 100 l) can be added to a daily bath or a coal tar medicated soap can be used. Alcoholic extract of tar (liquor picis carbonis) can be incorporated in an ointment, e.g. 2% to 6% in soft yellow paraffin. Coal tar paste B.P.C. can be used. Cleaner, washable proprietary tar creams are available e.g. Alphosyl (U.K.), Carbo Dome (U.K.) or Zetar℞ (U.S.A.). For the scalp coal tar and salicylic acid ointment B.P. is messy but extremely valuable as is Leeds Pomade (U.K.) which consists of 2% sulphur, 2% salicylic acid, 4% prepared coal tar, 25% emulsifying wax and liquid paraffin to 100%. The head is washed, initially daily, with a proprietary tar based shampoo e.g. Polytar (U.K.), Zetar℞,

(U.S.A.), or with 50% teepol and 1% glycerine in water. One popular regime, introduced 50 years ago by Goeckermann, is effective in most in-patients over 4 – 6 weeks and involves a daily tar bath, exposure to UVB, followed by application of a tar paste.

Dithranol (dihydroxyanthranol) (Anthralin[R], U.S.A.) is a more potent topical anti-mitotic but is more difficult to handle because it is an irritant to the unaffected skin. It is therefore incorporated in a concentration of 0.01% increasing to 0.5% in a stiff paste, zinc and salicylic acid paste B.P. (Lassar's paste). Dithranol stains linen permanently so the paste is applied once daily precisely to the lesions and then covered with tube gauze or an orthopaedic stockinette. The following day it is thoroughly removed in a tar bath, the patient exposed to UVB and the procedure repeated; this is the Ingram regime. Dithranol cannot be used on the face, ears, genitalia and flexures and is highly irritant if accidentally introduced into the eyes. In a suitably formulated pomade it can be used in the scalp. Efficient use of the Ingram regime for in-patients or out-patients attending a day-care centre will clear discoid psoriasis in most patients in about three weeks. A residual deep brown staining of the skin disappears within a month of the termination of treatment. The addition of UVB and the tar bath are not crucial. Dithranol is also available in an ointment base (Dithrolan, U.K.).

Corticosteroids are cleaner, non-irritant and much easier to use than tar or dithranol and are the treatment of choice for the face, ears, flexures and genitalia. However, prolonged use of the most potent preparations may destabilize the psoriasis, especially on withdrawal. Such preparations also induce cutaneous atrophy with consequent striae, telangiectasia, skin fragility and purpura. The rate of development and severity of these effects is proportional to the strength, quantities and duration of exposure. The face, flexures and backs of hands are particularly at risk. Widespread application of strong steroids in amounts exceeding 50 g per week may lead to Cushingoid features and hypothalamo-pituitary-adrenal suppression due to systemic absorption. Nevertheless, judiciously used corticosteroids have a valuable place in therapy. Lotions and gels of betamethasone valerate and fluocinolone acetonide are useful in the scalp. On the body, creams and ointments containing clobetasol propionate (Dermovate, U.K.), betamethasone valerate (Betnovate, U.K.; Valisone[R], U.S.A.), etc. can be applied once to thrice daily. For maintenance treatment medium strength preparations such as flurandrenolone (Cordran^R, U.S.A.) and hydrocortisone butyrate (Locoid, U.K.) are applicable.

Systemic treatment

When psoriasis is life-threatening or totally physically or socially disabling and either resistant to efficient topical therapy or relapses immediately after such treatment, methotrexate is the treatment of choice. This folate antagonist is given orally once weekly in a dose of 0.2 mg kg^{-1}, increasing if necessary to 0.4 mg kg^{-1}. It probably acts by inhibiting epidermal cell mitosis. Similar dosages can be administered *i.m.* or *i.v.* Response begins at two to three weeks and progresses for several weeks. Before treatment is begun it is essential to establish that renal, hepatic and marrow function are all normal. Alcoholism, active infection and a history of peptic ulceration are contra-indications. Maintenance treatment is effective and safe in experienced hands. Nausea lasting 24–36 hours is the commonest minor side-effect. The principal long term hazard is the development of hepatic fibrosis and even cirrhosis. Methotrexate is abortifacient and teratogenic and cannot be used in pregnancy.

Other cytostatic drugs sometimes of value include hydroxyurea (Hydrea, U.K.) and azathioprine (Imuran, U.K.)

Photochemotherapy

This is a new and highly effective form of treatment, apparently remarkably safe in the short term but whose long term efficacy and safety have yet to be established. It involves the oral administration of 8-methoxypsoralen, which is a photo-active coumarin compound of plant origin, followed two hours later by whole body exposure to a high potency source of long-wave ultra-violet light (UVA). The treatment is given thrice weekly initially and leads to steady clearance of psoriasis, together with development of a flattering tan. Maintenance treatment is needed once every 7–14 days to keep the psoriasis at bay. The theoretical long-term hazards include premature and accelerated ageing of the skin and carcinogenesis. For these reasons, the treatment is not yet approved and endorsed by the Committee on Safety of Medicines in the U.K. or by the Food and Drug Administration in the U.S.A.

19

LICHEN PLANUS

Lichen planus is an uncommon, but not rare, disease of the skin which runs a sub-acute or chronic course and has characteristic cutaneous and sometimes mucosal manifestations.

Aetiology

The cause of lichen planus is unknown. It may be exactly mimicked by certain drugs, suggesting the possibility that an unknown chemical toxin, perhaps in food, could be responsible. Claims have been made, on the basis of electron microscopic observations, that a virus is responsible but such claims are unconfirmed and do not satisfy Koch's postulates. Recent immunofluorescence studies suggest that autoimmune events in the region of the dermo-epidermal junction may be of importance.

Pathology

The histopathological features are those of an inflammatory 'attack' on the epidermis. The epidermis shows acanthosis, hyper-keratosis and prominence of the granular layer. There is patchy destruction of the basal epidermis with invasion by lymphocytes. The epidermo-dermal junction may assume a 'saw-tooth' pattern. Characteristically 'colloid' bodies, perhaps the 'ghosts' of des-troyed basal keratinocytes, are seen near the junction. In the papillary and sub-papillary dermis there is a dense band-like lympho-histiocytic infiltrate, which in the later stages contains many melanin-bearing macrophages.

The clinical picture

Lichen planus is one of the intensely pruritic skin diseases. It has a characteristic morphology which permits confident diagnosis on clinical grounds alone. The primary lesion is a 1–3 mm flat-topped papule with a shiny surface when viewed in reflected light. The papules have a characteristic red-purple hue. The surface of larger lesions is seen to be criss-crossed with fine white lines, called Wickham's striae (Plate IV). As the lesions enlarge and coalesce, flat topped plaques up to 2 cm in diameter may develop.

The sites of election are the flexor aspects of the wrists and forearms, the sides of the calves and ankles, the lower back and the shaft and glans of the penis, but lesions can appear anywhere.

Many morphological variants can occur. Lesions on the palms and soles are domed rather than flat and may be very hyperkeratotic. They may also have a pseudo-vesicular or even pseudo-pustular appearance. Grossly hypertrophic lesions up to 3 cm in diameter may occur on the legs, especially the anterior and lateral shins. Annular lesions with central clearing, sometimes atrophic, are seen, especially on the penis. Linear patterns may be due to trauma (Koebner phenomenon) or occur spontaneously. Follicular patterns, such as those seen in lichen plano-pilaris, may be confusing. Rarely a micro-papular form displays myriads of 1–2 mm papules especially on the trunk. In Africans a pityriasis rosea-like prodrome may be seen. Scalp involvement may result in rapidly progressive and irreversible scarring alopecia.

The nails are involved in about 10% of patients. The changes range from trivial flakiness of the surface of the nail plate, through longitudinal striations to marked thinning of the nail plate, koilonychial deformity or even complete destruction of the nails. Nail fold inflammation may be followed by atrophy and fusion of the posterior nail fold, nail bed and nail remnants (pterygium formation).

Mucous membrane involvement is frequent and usually affects the buccal mucosa (Fig. 82), lips or tongue. A lacy white network of papules on the buccal mucosa of the cheeks is most characteristic but areas of erythema, erosions, hypertrophic plaques and even ulceration may occur causing much discomfort.

Prognosis

Severe oral lichen planus and hypertrophic lichen of the legs may both be very intractable for many years or even decades. The ordinary disease usually lasts 6–24 months but is relapsing or chronic in a minority. As the lesions fade, hyperpigmentation remains and may take years to clear especially in coloured patients.

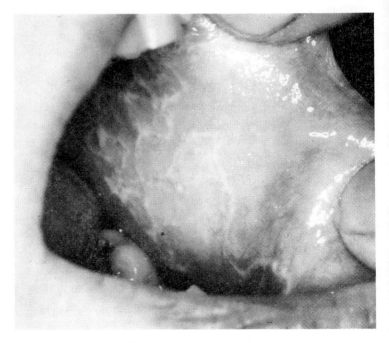

Fig. 82. Lichen planus on buccal mucosa.

Management

In very mild cases the disease can be ignored. If itching is trouble-some, topical steroids have to be used. Intra-lesional injection of steroid or a steroid-medicated adhesive tape are useful for hyper-trophic leg lesions. Betamethasone pellets are useful in severe oral forms. Intense pruritus may require oral administration of antihis-tamines and sedatives.

Rarely, steroids have to be used orally either because of the extent and severity of the itching and rash or because scalp involvement is threatening rapid and irreversible destruction of the hair follicles. Response to prednisolone 40 mg daily is usually excellent; the dose is quickly reduced to 20 mg daily and then slowly to zero by four months. A few patients cannot be managed without a small long-term maintenance dose.

Lichenoid Drug Eruption

Both the cutaneous and mucosal features of lichen planus may be induced by drugs. The picture may be pure as with mepacrine, chloroquine, amiphenazole and quinidine or mixed with eczematous or psoriasiform features as with gold and the abandoned beta-blocker, practolol. A lichenoid photo-dermatosis has been described in colour film processors. (See also Chapter 11.)

20

DISEASES OF INFANCY
AND CHILDHOOD

There is naturally a considerable overlap between childhood diseases and those of adult life, hence a number of the conditions mentioned here have also been dealt with in detail elsewhere in this book. Nevertheless it is of value to have a separate discussion of children's diseases, because knowing what diseases commonly occur in the young saves a good deal of time and enables a diagnosis to be made more speedily and accurately.

The skin of the new born may be bright red all over or may be mottled. Generalized peeling sometimes occurs. Lanugo hair may be profuse and the scalp hair may fall, to be replaced by the secondary terminal hairs. The skin is thin and permeable and substances such as hexachlorophane or boric acid applied topically can be absorbed into the blood system causing poisoning and even death. Strong undiluted steroids applied under the occlusion of a napkin can produce an alarming degree of atrophy. Under the influence of maternal hormones the sebaceous glands of the face may hypertrophy to produce pin-head pearly papules. The skin in older children can be quite hirsute if they are genetically predisposed but the hair is short or vellus in type. They may perspire very considerably. At puberty the secondary sexual hair appears and the sebaceous and the apocrine glands develop leading to greasiness and the aroma of the adult. School children are liable to infection in the process of building up immune responses. Those with infective processes, e.g. infected eczema and infection secondary to pediculosis capitis, may develop lymphadenopathy which lasts for some time but is essentially benign. Children develop many transient unexplained eruptions, most of which are probably responses to infection. Children develop allergic drug reactions and allergic contact dermatitis less frequently than adults.

Itching in infants is commonly due to scabies, eczema or

urticaria; in older children, insects bites and pediculosis should be
added to the list. Circinate eruptions in children may be due to
impetigo, which has a rapid onset and spread and is usually moist,
ringworm of the skin, which has a slower onset and is usually dry,
or granuloma annulare (see p. 184). Psoriasis in infants and children is most unusual but psoriasis-like napkin rashes which spread
are common.

The common neurotic traits in children affecting the skin are:
thumb and finger sucking which may lead to thickening of the skin
or to chronic paronychia, although some children develop chronic
paronychia for other reasons; hair pulling or rubbing leading to
localized alopecia; and lip licking, biting and sucking which cause
cheilitis and circumoral dermatitis. Psychogenic pruritus is rare
but the nervous child with atopic eczema experiences aggravation
of the itching and dermatitis in response to stress. A child may
refuse to attend school on account of a chronic non-infectious skin
disease. This requires special patience and understanding. The
head and the teachers of the school can often help in explaining the
non-infectious nature of the disease to the other pupils.

NAPKIN DERMATITIS

Cases of napkin dermatitis are exceedingly common; 40% commence in the first month and 90% in the first year of life. Most start
with a chemical burn either from contact with a stool or from
ammonia liberated from the urine in the napkins by urea-splitting
organisms. Infection often supervenes. A proportion are infective
especially in well-upholstered babies. Small disposable nappies
(Fig. 83) and the tight button-on type of plastic pants which go
with them predispose to irritation by concentrating the urine and
faeces in the manner of a patch test. The rash is usually erythematous and when produced by a stool burn is either peri-anal or
genital, or when produced by ammonia is on the convex surfaces.
Spread to the entire napkin area is common. It is not uncommon
for a seborrhoeic type of rash involving the scalp, face and axillae
to follow the development of a nappy rash. Secondary infection is
with faecal organisms, e.g. *Staphylococcus pyogenes* and *Candida albicans*.

Diagnosis. When localized to the nappy area there is no problem
in diagnosis; but disseminated cases are often wrongly labelled
infantile eczema. It is always wise to look at the napkin area in

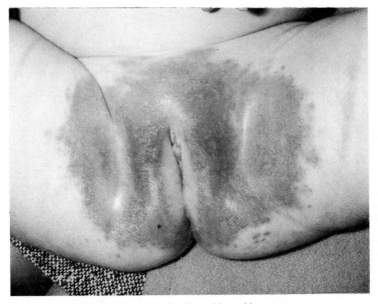

Fig. 83. Napkin rash: disposable napkin pattern.

babies with rashes and to ask whether the nappy rash preceded or
followed the rash elsewhere. Napkin rashes rarely irritate, whereas
infantile eczema always does. Some disseminated napkin rashes
look very like psoriasis, and may be called 'napkin psoriasis'.

Treatment. If it is feasible the napkins should be left off and the
infant allowed to lie on the napkin in a warm environment. Otherwise a non-wettable napkin (Marathon, U.K.) should be worn
next to the skin. This allows the urine to pass through it to a towel
napkin outside it. The plastic pants should be ample in size.
Napkins should be washed in soap flakes and if ammoniacal, be
given a final rinse in a vinegar in water solution, 50 ml in 5 l (1 fl oz
in 1 gal), or benzalkonium chloride 1:1000 (not boric acid which is
poisonous). An ointment should be applied to all affected areas e.g.
Tri-Adcortyl Ointment (U.K.) containing 0.1% triamcinolone acetonide, 0.25% neomycin sulphate, 0.025% gramicidin
and nystatin and 30 g soft paraffin to 150 g or Timodine (U.K.)
containing nystatin, hydrocortisone, benzalkonium chloride, and
silicone cream.

SEBORRHOEIC DERMATITIS

This is common in infancy. The commonest manifestation is the minimal one of scaling of the scalp, or milk crust. In other babies, especially those with deep folds, infective dermatitis of the neck fold, the axillae and groins may appear, overlapping disseminated napkin rash and giving a similar appearance. Sometimes infantile eczema may commence in the scalp and be erroneously labelled seborrhoeic dermatitis. Infantile eczema, however, always irritates, while seborrhoeic dermatitis rarely does.

Treatment. For 'milk crust' it is essential to wash the scalp daily with water, baby soap or baby shampoo; 0.5 per cent hydrocortisone ointment or 1% salicylic acid in emulsifying ointment (B.P.) should be applied. For the widespread type the ointment advised for napkin rash is advised for all affected areas including the scalp.

ALOPECIA

In babies the commonest cause of baldness is head rubbing. This may be a habit or it may be an attempt to alleviate the irritation of infantile eczema. In schoolchildren alopecia may be traumatic. Nervous children, especially girls, may pull out their own hair or twist or rub it so that it fractures. Sometimes a hank of hair is pulled out by another child. Alopecia areata is also common in childhood and ringworm of the scalp must not be forgotten.

SCALY PATCHES OF CHILDHOOD

Scaly patches are very common from late infancy to the late teens and may also occur in adult life. The exposed parts are affected, especially the face. One appearance is of scaling with or without erythema. If the skin is pigmented a white appearance results, hence the name pityriasis alba. In spite of the other name for this condition, impetigo pityroides, no organism can be consistently recovered and the aetiology is obscure. A naturally dry skin plus non-specific traumata such as sun, wind, cold and soap may be responsible.

The response to treatment is unsatisfactory. Stopping the use of soap to the face or affected area and the use of a greasy ointment, e.g. soft yellow paraffin with or without 0.25% oxytetracycline, may be helpful. Scaly patches which irritate may be a minimal form of atopic eczema and can be helped by the application of 1 % hydrocortisone.

Urticaria

Urticaria in children is often easier to deal with than in adults. Children with atopic eczema who develop urticaria are often sensitive to a specific food. Note that exacerbations of the urticaria following challenge with the appropriate food do not affect the eczema. Other children develop acute urticaria which lasts a few days or a few weeks; this type is probably due to an infection. Cold urticaria is not infrequent, but heat urticaria is rarer.

Papular urticaria is usually a response to insect bites. The first time a particular insect bites a child there is no response but later bites may excite an immunological reaction which is urticarial or even vesicular or bullous. In the course of time spontaneous desensitization may occur.

Other Diseases of Infancy

Infantile eczema is a common complaint which usually begins between the ages of two to six months. It affects the face, scalp, knee flexures, elbows and sometimes the hands and trunk. It is always irritating. (See also p. 125.)

Scabies is another very irritating disease of infants. As well as affecting the usual adult sites, it often affects the soles of the feet and sometimes the face of babies. (See also p. 100.)

Impetigo is very common in schoolchildren. (See p. 48.)

Naevi or birthmarks are discussed on pages 218 and 238.

Acne frequently occurs in infants.

21

TUMOURS

BENIGN EPIDERMAL TUMOURS AND CYSTS

BASAL CELL PAPILLOMA

These lesions, also called seborrhoeic warts, seborrhoeic keratosis, and senile warts, are almost universal in the second half of life. They develop in both sexes particularly on the upper trunk, brow, temples and face. The lesions are grey-brown, brown or almost black and often have a greasy appearance (Fig. 84). They are

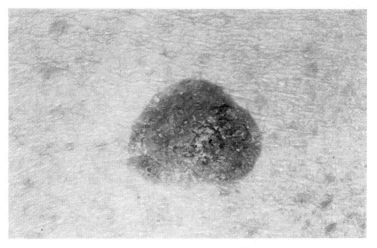

Fig. 84. Basal cell papilloma (seborrhoeic wart). Note 'stuck-on' appearance.

round or ovoid and may reach diameters measuring up to 3 or 4 cm. They may be almost flat or raised, sessile nodules or even pedunculated. The surface is irregular and papillomatous in bigger lesions.

Differential diagnosis is from moles, pigmented basal cell carcinoma, lentigo maligna and malignant melanoma.

Cryotherapy with liquid nitrogen is effective. Very large and numerous lesions are best curetted off flush with the skin surface. Local anaesthesia is often unnecessary. Very light galvano-cautery or oxycel dressings suffice for haemostasis. Healing is rapid and should leave little scarring.

SQUAMOUS PAPILLOMA

Solitary wart-like papillomata are sometimes seen in the elderly, usually on the face. They rarely grow larger than 5–7 mm. They can be destroyed by liquid nitrogen or curetted out and cauterized under local anaesthesia.

CLEAR CELL ACANTHOMA

This is a very rare solitary nodule, also called Degos acanthoma, which develops slowly over many years or even decades, usually on a leg. Its surfaces may be scaly or look eroded or translucent. Histologically, the acanthotic epidermis shows characteristic areas of 'clear' cells which contain glycogen. Excision-biopsy is the treatment.

EPIDERMAL CYSTS

These are commonly misnamed 'sebaceous cysts'. Epidermal cysts are of two types, epidermoid and pilar. Epidermoid cysts can occur on any part of the body. They present as firm swellings with a smooth overlying epidermis usually showing a central punctum. The cyst contains keratin, not sebum, produced by the epithelial lining which shows normal maturation, including granular layer formation. Surgical excision is the treatment of choice. Epidermoid cysts are associated with intestinal polyposis in Gardner's syndrome which is inherited in an autosomal dominant fashion. Malignant transformation of the polyps is not uncommon. Pilar (wen; tricholemmal) cysts are usually multiple and occur on the scalp. They may be familial. The cyst is tense, smooth and does not show a punctum. Its epithelial lining resembles the outer root sheath of hair follicles. The contents are keratinous but a granular layer does not form. Treatment is by excision.

Milia are pinhead epidermoid cysts commonly seen on the upper cheeks and around the eyes in young adults. Each milium is seen as a glistening white 1–2 mm papule which can be lifted out with the point of a sterile hypodermic needle. The development of milia may be secondary to trauma and inflammation, particularly following sub-epidermal blistering. Such milia are seen in the scars of epidermolysis bullosa dystrophica, bullous pemphigoid and porphyria cutanea tarda.

INTERMEDIATE EPIDERMAL TUMOURS

ACTINIC KERATOSIS

These lesions, also called solar keratosis and solar keratoma, are usually multiple and occur on exposed skin. Their development and number are directly proportional to the fairness of the patient's skin, his age, and the amount and intensity of sunlight to which the skin has been exposed. The lesions are palpable, scaly, rough to the touch and often brownish in colour. The scale is adherent. The lesion is usually discrete but after decades of gross sun exposure virtually the whole of the exposed skin may be dyskeratotic (Fig. 8).

Squamous cell carcinomata may slowly develop in a very small proportion but are not usually aggressive, i.e. metastasis is slow.

Treatment requires experience and expertise. Controlled topical application of 1% to 5% 5-fluorouracil lotion or cream is the treatment of choice but cryotherapy, curettage and even dermabrasion of localized lesions have their place.

BOWEN'S DISEASE

Bowen's disease, or intra-epidermal carcinoma, is an uncommon, usually solitary, condition seen in the second half of life. It can occur anywhere on the body. Usually it develops *de novo* but may be caused by solar damage, X-irradiation and previous oral therapy with inorganic arsenic.

The lesion presents as a psoriasis-like or eczema-like plaque, spreading very slowly over many years and with a characteristically irregular contour. Its diameter may be several centimetres. It is fixed, scaly or crusted and quite unresponsive to topical steroids. Itching is usually minimal. Evolution into invasive squamous cell carcinoma is very unusual.

The diagnosis is confirmed by biopsy. Surgical excision is the treatment of choice but cryotherapy, radiotherapy or curettage may be more appropriate in some cases.

Erythroplasia of Queyrat is Bowen's disease occurring on the penis. It is commoner in the uncircumcized and usually straddles the glans and distal shaft. After biopsy confirmation, radiotherapy is the treatment of choice. Differential diagnosis is from psoriasis, lichen planus and plasma cell balanitis of Zoon.

PAGET'S DISEASE OF THE BREAST

In this rare disease an eczema-like eruption develops in the skin of the nipple and slowly spreads centrifugally on the breast (Fig. 85). The surface of the plaque is moist and crusted and the disease is unresponsive to topical corticosteroids. Differential diagnosis is from eczema and is confirmed by biopsy which reveals metastatic Paget's cells in the epidermis. These are malignant cells arising

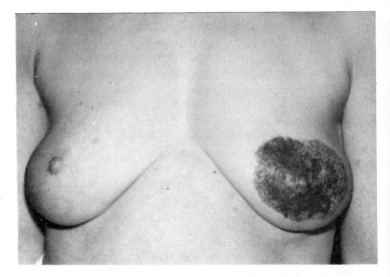

Fig. 85. Paget's disease of breast (advanced).

from an underlying intraductal carcinoma of the breast. The treatment is mastectomy.

Extra-mammary Paget's disease

This rare condition arises from the adnexal apocrine structures and occurs in the ano-genital region or axilla. Underlying carcinoma must be excluded.

CUTANEOUS HORN

This is a rare lesion seen in old people. A warty papule slowly develops a horn-like hyperkeratotic extension which may reach 2 cm or more in length. The base is indurated and may be the seat of a low grade squamous cell carcinoma. Complete excision is advised.

KERATO-ACANTHOMA

Kerato-acanthoma, or molluscum sebaceum, is a rapidly growing but self healing tumour thought to arise from a hair follicle. The tumour is generally solitary and favours the face or arm. A rapidly growing papule matures in a few weeks into a domed firm nodule up to 2 cm in diameter. As the lesion develops its sides show a bulging convexity and its crown may have a whitish appearance with a central horny plug (Plate VII). The nodule reaches its maximum size by eight weeks, then remains stationary for weeks or months before involuting (if left untouched), often leaving a depressed scar.

Curettage in one piece is the treatment of choice and also provides adequate histological material. Under low power magnification the architecture is characteristic but the cytology of a rapidly growing lesion in a small biopsy may be impossible to distinguish from that of squamous cell carcinoma. Occasionally lesions recur after curettage and may cause anxiety. Rarely tumours clinically and histologically indistinguishable from kerato-acanthoma subsequently behave as metastasizing squamous cell carcinomata.

LEUKOPLAKIA

This is a particular pattern of hyperplasia of skin or mucous membranes characterized clinically by the formation of thickened, whitish-grey, well-defined plaques and histologically by hyper-keratosis and acanthosis with dysplasia of the epidermal cells. It may proceed to squamous cell carcinoma. It is seen in the second half of life and external irritants play a role in its development. It is seen in the mouth or the lip, buccal mucosa or tongue. It is also seen in the ano-genital region in women. In oral leukoplakia, pipe smoking, ill-fitting dentures or abnormal teeth may be responsible. In.genital lesions, discharges, maceration and friction may be relevant.

In the mouth differential diagnosis is from simple mucosal hyperplasia due to gum biting and chewing, lichen planus and white sponge naevus. Ano-genital leukoplakia must be differenti-ated from lichen sclerosus et atrophicus and from lichenified eczema or psoriasis.

Histologically unequivocal lesions should be excised surgically. Irritant factors must be removed.

MALIGNANT EPIDERMAL TUMOURS

BASAL CELL CARCINOMA

A basal cell carcinoma, or rodent ulcer, is a slow growing, locally malignant growth usually arising during middle or old age, and is usually found on the face. Men are more frequently affected than women.

Basal cell carcinoma consists of an agglomeration of small com-pact cells, with deeply staining nuclei, which grow down from the basal layers of the epidermis or from the similar cell layers of the hair follicle. These cells grow into the dermis in irregular columns. The columns are confined and localized by a palisade layer of columnar cells, which have a rudimentary resemblance to the columnar cells of the basal cell layer. These tumours are not therefore metastatic, for, so long as the line of columnar cells remains unbroken, metastases cannot form in adjacent or remote organs; but they are locally malignant, for the cells invade con-tiguous tissue, including cartilage and bone. It should be noted that 'cell nests' are not found. As the tumours are relatively avascu-lar, necrosis and ulceration of the central areas occur easily.

There are three clinical types of basal cell carcinoma:

1. Simple, which in the early stages is a small, slow growing tumour.

2. Morphoea-like or card-like type which spreads laterally, forming a plaque without invasion of the deeper tissues.

3. Cystic, in which colloid degeneration occurs and cysts are formed which contain a gelatinous fluid.

Usually the lesion commences as a small, hard, painless, superficial nodule which, during a course of from eighteen months to three years, enlarges until it becomes about a centimetre in diameter, and necroses in the centre. At this stage it has a hard, raised, pearly telangiectatic edge which forms the rim of the crateriform ulcer (Fig. 86), the centre of which is covered by a

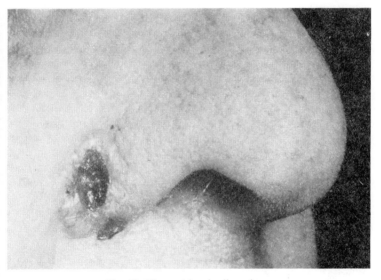

Fig. 86. Ulcerated basal cell carcinoma.

brownish crust. When the crust is removed a reddish area of pseudo-granulation tissue is exposed. The lesion is invariably circular or oval. If left untreated the growth erodes the deeper tissues, and once the underlying bone is involved the condition may be incurable. In the later stages the eye may be destroyed or an antrum laid open by the relentless progress of the tumour.

The morphoea-like basal cell carcinoma spreads slowly across the skin. Its edge is raised, but behind the advancing periphery the skin is smooth, flattened, ivory-like and resembles an area of scleroderma. A few small ulcers may appear on the surface of the plaque, but ulceration is not a feature of the malady. This form of carcinoma produces a considerable fibrous reaction which may cause atrophy of the cancerous cells and thus cause partial healing.

The cystic variety is a soft, bluish-white, semi-translucent cyst, varying in diameter from a few millimetres to about 2 cm in diameter. Small blood vessels can usually be seen coursing over it.

Basal cell carcinomata may be very pigmented and hence need to be distinguished from melanomata.

Treatment may be by excision or by radiotherapy. For lesions less than 1 cm in size excellent results are obtained by curettage and cauterization in skilled hands. Morphoea-like carcinomata should be treated by excision and grafting; they are insensitive to radiotherapy.

Squamous Cell Carcinoma

These malignant growths are capable of metastasizing, usually via the lymphatic channels. The face and the mucous membrane of the lips are the sites of election, i.e. sun-exposed areas, but these tumours may be found elsewhere on the body and on the extremities; for example, they may arise from areas of actinic keratosis (see p. 210) or develop on the tongue or within the vagina or balano-preputial sac. In some cases one can obtain a history of long-continued exposure of the affected area to chemical or physical irritants. X-ray workers used to frequently develop squamous carcinomata on the hands, as did persons who were continually exposed to tar or paraffin. These industrial hazards have now been overcome to a large degree by adequate protective and preventive measures. Pipe smokers, especially those who use clay pipes, may develop the tumour on the lip or tongue. Tar workers may develop the disease. Machine operators develop epithelioma of the scrotum through the irritation of heavy oils, and it is the duty of employers to warn these people of the dangers, to advise precautions and to provide six-monthly medical examinations.

More cases are seen in males than in females. Squamous carcinomata are seldom seen in persons under 45 years of age.

Pathologically, the tumours are found to consist of irregular branching columns of epithelial cells which pass inwards from the epidermis and may penetrate the subjacent tissues to a considerable depth. The cells of the tumour resemble prickle cells, being large and polygonal, often with definite fibrils bridging the intercellular spaces. At the growing edges of the tumour embryonic and primitive types of cells are found. A characteristic feature, which is not always present, is the formation of cell nests. These are formed of concentric layers of keratinized cells, which stain deeply. Surrounding the keratinized cells are layers of uncornified cells. The more numerous the cell nests, the less dangerous is the neoplasm.

Macroscopically the tumour commences as a nodule which grows fairly rapidly and forms an oval or circular tumour, raised a few millimetres above the level of the surrounding skin (Fig. 87).

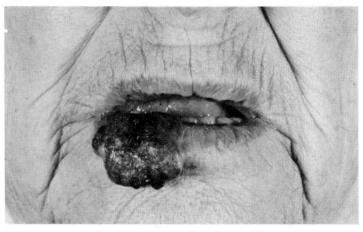

Fig. 87. Squamous cell carcinoma of lip.

Ulceration may occur and the edges of the fully-formed lesion are everted. If left untreated, a fungating tumour develops and erodes all the adjacent tissues; metastases form in the proximal lymphatic glands, and may occur in distant organs.

Treatment should consist of excision, radiotherapy or a mixture of the two, according to size, site, age of patient, etc.

Malignant melanoma (See p. 239.)

BENIGN TUMOURS OF THE DERMIS

HISTIOCYTOMA (DERMATOFIBROMA)

These are common lesions, more often seen in females particularly in middle life and usually on the legs. They may be solitary or multiple and are generally symptomless. The clinical features are quite characteristic, revealing a small 5–10 mm hard papule or nodule, often rather flat and with a 'button-like' shape on palpation. The lesion is firmly attached to skin and its surface is bound down. The colour is usually a pale or deeper yellow-brown. It grows very slowly and then remains stationary for years.

Histologically, a well circumscribed mass of connective tissue cells is seen in the dermis. Often the overlying epidermis shows modest basaloid hyperplasia.

Treatment, when requested, is excision.

GRANULOMA TELANGIECTATICUM

This common lesion, also 'called pyogenic granuloma, usually occurs at sites of trauma and is seen on the fingers or face. It presents as a rapidly growing friable papule which bleeds easily. Large lesions may reach a diameter of 10 – 15 mm and become pedunculated. More often the lesion sits in a ring of sodden epithelium like an acorn in its cup. Long-lasting lesions grow a surface epithelium and become less friable. Histologically a mass of proliferative small blood vessels is set in a stroma infiltrated with inflammatory cells.

Curettage and cauterization is the best treatment but cryotherapy is often effective.

SPIDER NAEVUS

In this congenitally determined lesion a dilated arteriole produces a tiny red papule. Branching tributaries form 'spider's legs'. Some young people have a few spider naevi which are found on the head, neck or upper limbs. The spider naevi may appear during pregnancy, only to resolve promptly in the puerperium. In other circumstances, the presence of large numbers of lesions raises suspicion of chronic liver disease.

Spider naevi must be distinguished from venous 'stars', cherry angiomata (Campbell de Morgan spots) and the telangiectatic lesions of Osler's disease and systemic sclerosis.

Cauterization of the central arteriole is effective treatment.

CAPILLARY HAEMANGIOMA

Capillary haemangioma, or port-wine stain, is a developmental defect rather than a tumour. The lesion is present at birth and never disappears. It is usually unilateral and appears initially as a wine-coloured macular lesion, usually on one side of the face. Histologically a mass of abnormal dilated vessels occupies the superficial dermis. In later life the lesion may become proliferative and nodular.

Treatment is palliative. Cosmetic covering may be all that is possible but cryotherapy and later plastic surgery have a very limited place.

CAVERNOUS HAEMANGIOMA

The commonest lesion of this type is the 'strawberry naevus'. This is not present at birth but is first seen a few weeks later as a red papule which grows rapidly (Fig. 88). The fully mature lesion is reached by the age of six months and may be tiny or enormous. Lesions in the napkin area may ulcerate or bleed. Those on the face may interfere with the establishment of binocular vision. Rarely, massive 'tumours' sequestrate platelets leading to thrombocytopenia and purpura. After several months spontaneous involution begins, evident as whitish zones within the lesion. Over many years involution is complete leaving minimal cosmetic defect.

Management is always conservative where possible. A series of photographs showing involution provides useful reassurance for parents. Radiotherapy, cryotherapy and surgery should be avoided as they worsen the cosmetic prognosis.

HAEMANGIOMA SIMPLEX

Simple haemangiomata may develop in later life. The lower lip is probably the commonest site. Small lesions can be destroyed by electro-cautery but larger ones should be excised.

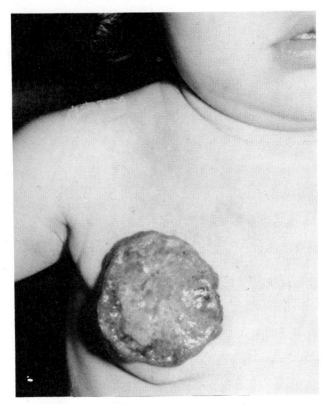

Fig. 88. Ulcerated cavernous haemangioma.

GLOMANGIOMA

This tumour arises from the glomus body of the dermis, which is a specialized arterio-venous shunt by-passing the papillary capillaries. The central canal is lined by glomus cells derived from smooth muscle.

The glomus tumour is usually a solitary blue-red soft papule which is tender on compression and which may be spontaneously painful. It is generally found peripherally on a limb and may occur on the nail bed. The treatment is surgical excision.

Neurofibromatosis. (See p. 42.)

MALIGNANT TUMOURS OF THE DERMIS

SECONDARY DEPOSITS

The skin may be the seat of metastatic deposits from an internal carcinoma. The breast is the usual primary site but tumours of the gastro-intestinal tract and bronchus are occasionally responsible. The lesions are usually multiple painless hard nodules in the dermis and sub-cutis. The diagnosis is confirmed by biopsy.

KAPOSI'S SARCOMA

This is a rare tumour of elderly men, also called idiopathic haemorrhagic sarcoma, is classically described in eastern European Jews but now known to occur throughout the world and to be particularly common in parts of Africa. Multiple blue-red warty nodules usually begin on the skin of the feet and slowly spread to the legs. Later the disease causes increasing oedema of the lower limbs due to lymphatic obstruction and may spread to the lymph glands and systemic organs. It is a tumour of multicentric origin with vascular endothelial and fibroblastic elements. After a course of up to 10 years, it is eventually fatal.

ANGIOSARCOMA

Malignant angio-endothelioma is a rare tumour, usually seen on the head in the elderly arising in cutaneous blood vessels.

MYCOSIS FUNGOIDES AND SEZARY SYNDROME

Mycosis fungoides is an uncommon malignant proliferation of lymphoid tissue, affecting principally lymphocytes of T lineage. It is a particularly dermotropic tumour, usually confined to the skin for years or even decades and only involving glands and internal organs at a late stage. Three clinical stages are described. In the first, which may last for many years, apparently non-specific inflammation may simulate eczema or psoriasis. Later, in stage 2, the lesions become more infiltrated and may be bizarre in contour (Fig. 89). In the final stage, frank tumours appear and may ulcerate. Itching may be severe. Because the bone marrow is not involved, the patient is not anaemic.

One variant can produce a generalized exfoliative dermatitis or a bright, universal erythroderma. In the latter type, characteristic neoplastic T-cells can be found in the peripheral blood (Sezary syndrome). A T-cell leukaemia may supervene.

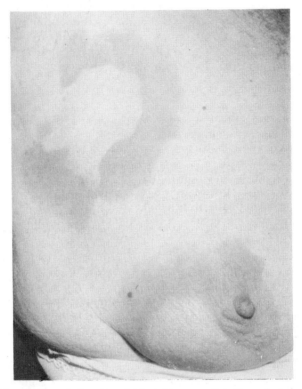

Fig. 89. Mycosis fungoides: infiltrated tumours. Note 'horse shoe' shape.

Other lympho-reticular malignancies, such as lymphosarcoma, Hodgkin's disease, reticulum cell sarcoma and various leukaemias may infiltrate the skin. The non-specific manifestations of these diseases are described in Chapter 23.

22

CUTANEOUS MANIFESTATIONS OF MALIGNANT DISEASE

The skin may be involved in systemic malignant disease specifically and non-specifically. Specific involvement means actual neoplastic infiltration of the skin by secondary deposits from an internal carcinoma, such as from the breast, or by deposits of a reticulo-endothelial malignancy such as leukaemia, lymphosarcoma, mycosis fungoides, or even, though rarely, Hodgkin's disease. Morphologically such lesions are likely to be papules, nodules, plaques or tumours involving mainly the dermis but often with epidermal involvement, as in the case of the lymphomata. The diagnosis is established without difficulty by biopsy.

In contrast, there is no histological evidence of malignant cells in the skin in the non-specific reactions. Clinical experience has demonstrated the importance of a number of cutaneous reactions which are sometimes called 'markers' of malignancy. Their presence calls for further investigation in search of a carcinoma or lymphoma. The mechanisms by which these markers develop are barely understood but immunological factors are thought to play a role in some.

The non-specific markers are best sub-divided into three groups as follows:
1. Those almost always associated with malignancy.
2. Those sometimes associated with malignancy.
3. Those suggestive of reticulo-endothelial malignancy.

CONDITIONS ALMOST ALWAYS ASSOCIATED WITH MALIGNANCY

Paget's disease

This epidermal tumour of the breast simulating eczema is always due to an underlying ductal carcinoma of the breast tissue. (See p. 213.)

Acanthosis nigricans

This rare but distinctive condition develops *de novo* in the second half of life in subjects who are not obese and, in the absence of endocrinopathy, indicates an internal malignancy, usually a carcinoma in the gastrointestinal tract, especially the stomach. The cutaneous changes may herald the appearance of a detectable tumour or the latter may be well established by the time skin changes are seen.

The cutaneous changes consist of epidermal thickening and hyperpigmentation particularly in the flexures and neck. The affected skin may become velvety but patchy wartiness is common. The palms and soles may be involved.

Milder similar changes may be seen in obese adolescents particularly of dark skinned ethnic groups such as Arabs and Indians, especially in the axillae and around the neck. Certain endocrinopathies in children may also be associated with similar changes, sometimes called pseudo-acanthosis nigricans and of no sinister significance.

Erythema gyratum repens

This is a very rare but distinctive pattern of erythema in which concentric erythematous rings and wavy patterns are closely packed over the whole body. The patterns change visibly day by day leaving scaling on the trailing edge of the waves of erythema. The condition may convert to a universal erythroderma. A carcinoma is always present eventually, often of the bronchus.

Necrolytic migratory erythema

This is an equally rare but morphologically and histologically distinctive eruption associated with weight loss and angular stomatitis. Its presence indicates the existence of a glucagon-secreting tumour, usually malignant, of the α-islet cells of the pancreas.

CONDITIONS SOMETIMES ASSOCIATED WITH MALIGNANCY

Dermatomyositis

This syndrome is described on page 170. Cutaneous changes may be absent as in carcinomatous polymyositis or the skin changes may predominate or precede myositis by weeks or months. It is the least rare of the 'collagen' diseases in childhood, when it has no malignant implications, but in patients over 40 years, about one third have or will develop a tumour.

Multicentric reticulohistiocytosis

This is a rare disease of skin and joints, which usually occurs in women, in which a mutilating and destructive arthritis of peripheral joints is associated with a characteristic eruption of reddish-yellow papules and nodules particularly on the face, shoulders and upper limbs. 'Coral bead' papules around the nail folds are distinctive. About 25% of patients with multicentric reticulohistiocytosis develop a carcinoma.

Atypical bullous pemphigoid

A number of instances have been reported in which atypical bullous eruptions, most closely resembling bullous pemphigoid, have been associated with an internal tumour. The possibility should be borne in mind when atypical clinical, histological or immunofluorescence findings occur in bullous diseases.

Peutz-Jegher syndrome

This genetically determined syndrome features gastrointestinal polyps. Those in the stomach or colon may undergo malignant transformation. Pigmentation of the lips is a constant feature.

Gardner's syndrome

In this rare condition, multiple subcutaneous epidermoid cysts are associated with osseous lesions and polyposis of the colon which can become carcinomatous.

Keratoderma of palms and soles

A very small number of families has been described in which hereditary tylosis is associated with a strong tendency to premature (second and third decade) development of carcinoma of the oesophagus.

CONDITIONS SUGGESTIVE OF RETICULO-ENDOTHELIAL MALIGNANCY

Pigmentation

Marked pigmentation is not uncommon in malignant cachexia. It may be associated with generalized pruritus in Hodgkin's disease. The groins, nipples and axillae are most often involved.

Pruritus

In middle age intractable generalized itching, in the absence of the well known causes such as skin diseases and infestation, liver and renal disease, may herald a lymphoma, particularly Hodgkin's disease. Pruritus may also be associated with a carcinoma, e.g. of the stomach. It should be remembered that in old age itching associated with dryness of the skin is common, especially in men.

Acquired ichthyosis

Ichthyosis is usually genetically determined and present from infancy. Appearing for the first time in middle or late life it may have sinister implications of lymphomatous disease. The histological features are non-specific.

Poikiloderma atrophicans vasculare

The combination of atrophy of the skin, patchy pigmentation and telangiectasia is seen in sun-damaged skin and after radiotherapy. Occurring *de novo* on covered areas it is a feature of lymphomata. Widespread forms of poikiloderma may develop into mycosis fungoides. Localized forms may be associated with reticulum cell sarcoma or lymphosarcoma.

Erythroderma

Universal inflammation of the skin, sometimes called generalized exfoliative dermatitis, has been discussed as a complication of psoriasis (p. 194) or eczema (p. 141) and as a drug-induced phenomenon (p. 147). It may also be associated with a malignant lymphoma either as a presenting feature or during the course of the illness. In such circumstances, the erythroderma is intractable. Although the histology is non-specific at first, the inflamed skin may eventually become infiltrated with lymphomatous cells.

Drug-induced changes

Lastly, although drug-induced changes are described elsewhere, it should be mentioned that cutaneous evidence of previous administration of inorganic arsenic, e.g. palmar keratoses, rain-drop pigmentation, or the presence of intraepidermal (Bowen's) or basal cell carcinomata implies an increased risk of internal carcinoma, especially of the bronchus.

23

PSYCHOGENIC DISORDERS

The concept of psychosomatic disease is well established. It can apply to many organs and is widely believed to be particularly important in skin disease. The solid evidence that this is so appears less convincing and the mechanisms, other than autonomic ones, are not understood. However, on the basis of such obvious phenomena as flushing induced by embarrassment, pallor due to fear or anger, the ability of emotions to influence the skin is accepted, particularly by the lay mind. The following discussion will be confined to those few clinical situations where the psychic disorder unequivocally underlies cutaneous symptoms or signs.

Psychogenic pruritus

Pruritus, generalized or localized, may on occasion be entirely psychogenic in origin and due either to anxiety or depression. The symptoms may be acute or chronic. The scalp is a favourite site for localization. Physical signs may be absent or there may be scratch marks, frictional erythema or lichenified nodules.

Other causes of pruritus, particularly cutaneous infection and systemic organic disease, must be excluded with certainty. Treatment must be directed to the underlying emotional disorder. Topical anti-pruritics are of little value.

Delusions of parasitism

Psychotic subjects with various forms of schizophrenia and paranoia may have unshakeable delusions that insects are crawling in or under the skin. Such patients complain of itching and may produce tiny fragments of dirt, hair or stratum corneum as evidence of such infestation. This is a rare condition and has to be distinguished from the more common symptom, formication, where the patient has a sensation 'as though insects are crawling in the skin' but is prepared to accept the doctor's statement after examination that this is not so.

Acne excoriée

It is not uncommon for adolescent girls or young women with or without acne vulgaris to have an irresistible desire to pick at and excoriate 'spots' on the face. The resultant lesions are characteristic artefactual erosions which may leave scarring. There seems to be a strong correlation between the presence of this condition and obvious emotional disturbance.

Control of the acne may help the situation but treatment can be very difficult and psychiatric help may be needed.

Cholinergic urticaria

This is a common pattern of urticaria characterized by the development of numerous pin-head weals surrounded by large erythematous flares and precipitated by heat, exercise and particularly emotional stress. It is relatively unresponsive to antihistamines but eventually undergoes spontaneous remission. (See p. 153.)

Dermatitis artefacta

Dermatitis artefacta is a self-inflicted inflammation or injury of the skin. The lesions occur on any part of the body which the patient's hands can reach easily. If the patient is right-handed, there are usually more lesions on the left side of the body, and *vice versa*. The types of lesions usually encountered are deep excoriations of the skin caused by scratching, or various erythemata caused by the application of easily obtainable rubefacients, e.g. mustard.

Many of the patients show a pernicious ingenuity in the manufacture of lesions, and unless the physician is very alert he may fail to diagnose the 'disease'. The lesions are bizarre in character and shape and, in some cases of exceptional severity, with deep excoriations and ulcerations (Fig. 90).

Dermatitis artefacta is in many cases a symptom of hysteria. Occasionally, non-hysterical subjects resort to self-inflicted lesions in order to evade work or obtain compensation. The majority of cases occur in young women.

Diagnosis may be difficult. Very close observation, especially in

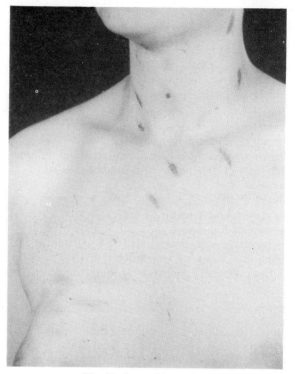

Fig. 90. Dermatitis artefacta.

hospital, may establish that lesions appear suddenly, e.g. over-night. A search of the patient's bedside locker may reveal the weapon employed. Occlusion of lesions on a limb by means of zinc paste bandage, B.P.C. or plaster of Paris will allow rapid healing.

Neurotic excoriations

Some patients present with deep excoriations on parts of the body accessible to the finger nails. The consistent absence of primary lesions which have not been scratched is a diagnostic feature. Psychiatric assessment usually reveals an underlying emotional problem. Treatment is often ineffective, and the resources of the psychiatrist, social worker and family usually have to be harnessed.

Hair pulling and rubbing

The habit of twisting a lock of hair and so producing a patch of alopecia is common in nervous children. Recovery is usually spontaneous. Perpetual rubbing of the hair resulting in uniformly short fractured hairs is a symptom of a more deep seated psychiatric disorder. (See also p. 252.)

24

DISORDERS OF PIGMENTATION

The normal skin owes its pigmentation to the yellow, brown or black pigment, melanin. The amount of melanin present depends on the race and on the degree of exposure to sunlight. Melanin is produced from tyrosine under the influence of tyrosinase in the melanocyte. The compound is attached to protein, forming melanoprotein. The melanocytes are cells derived from the neural crest which migrate in foetal life and attach themselves to the basal cell layer of the epidermis. The melanocyte secretes the pigment, melanin, into the cells of the epidermis, and protects against ultra-violet light. Hence negroes rarely develop cancer of the epidermis, yet curiously enough they have no more melanocytes than do white Caucasians; the negro melanocyte, however, produces far more melanin.

HYPOPIGMENTATION

Melanocyte stimulating hormone, ACTH, oestrogen and progesterone stimulate melanogenesis. In *panhypopituitarism* the lack of these hormones causes the skin to be pale in colour. The term leucoderma means abnormally white skin, usually localized in patches.

Albinism

Albinism, or oculocutaneous albinism, is an autosomal recessive condition in which melanin is not produced although the number of melanocytes is normal. These individuals have blond hair and fair skin. The presence of nystagmus provides a clue to the diagnosis. Pink eyes are rare in human albinos.

Piebaldism

Piebaldism is of autosomal dominant transmission and presents at birth with white patches of skin and a white forelock. The melano-cytes are missing from the white areas. If other defects are present including deafness, the diagnosis of Waardenburg's syndrome should be considered.

Phenylketonuria

Phenylketonuria is an inborn error of phenylalanine metabolism. The hair and skin are fair and the eyes are blue. Darkening occurs on a low phenylalanine diet. Eczema is frequent in these individuals.

Vitiligo

Vitiligo is the commonest type of leucoderma (Fig. 91). White patches appear in childhood or adult life. The face, the backs of the hands, the axillae and the perineum are the common sites. The surrounding skin may appear more darkly pigmented than nor-mal. Vitiligo in whites may be invisible in the winter. In coloured people vitiligo is a great embarrassment and cause for concern. The melanocytes are either absent or very much diminished in number. The latest hypothesis is that an autoimmune inflamma-tion destroys the pigment cells. Evidence for this view is largely indirect: the fact that organ-specific antibodies and organ-specific autoimmune diseases such as diabetes, hypothyroidism, and Addisonian anaemia are statistically commoner in vitiligo patients than in controls.

The treatment of vitiligo is not very satisfactory although suc-cess has been claimed with the strong local steroid ointments and creams that are now being used. Prolonged treatment is required. Trimethylpsoralen or 8-methoxypsoralen have been used either by mouth or applied locally and followed by exposure to longwave ultra-violet light (UVA) but the success rate is low. Cosmetic camouflage creams are very useful, especially in females.

Chemically-induced hypopigmentation

Hydroquinones may inhibit melanogenesis and even destroy melanocytes, and patients with white patches should therefore be asked if they are in contact with chemicals. Photographers use hydroquinone. Tertiary butyl phenols which are used in disinfec-tants and glues also produce depigmentation. Chemical workers may be in contact with both types of compound. It has recently

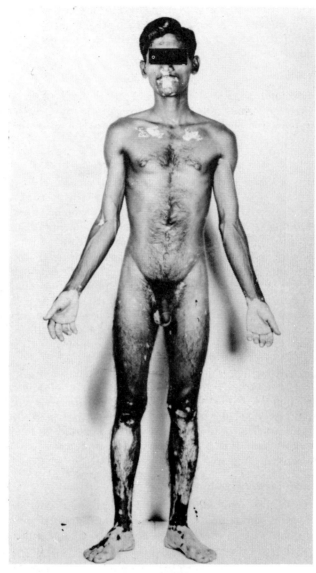

Fig. 91. Vitiligo.

been discovered that the whitish patches occurring on tanned or dark skin in tinea versicolor infections are the result of the inhibition of melanin synthesis by a chemical secreted by the fungus (Fig. 92).

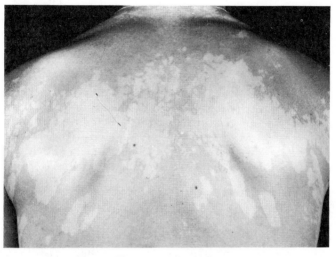

Fig. 92. Tinea versicolor: depigmentation.

Other causes of hypopigmentation

Another infection which produces whitish patches is leprosy, where the patches are usually hypaesthetic (see Chapter 5). Ash leaf-shaped white patches present at birth are a marker of the genetic disease tuberose sclerosis (see Chapter 4). Inflammation of the skin, especially dark skin, often produces temporary depigmentation, e.g. psoriasis and eczema (Figs. 93 and 94). Scarring processes may produce permanent white areas, e.g. trauma, burns, and discoid lupus erythematosus.

HYPERPIGMENTATION

Excess of MSH or ACTH produces hyperpigmentation. *Addison's disease* is a good example of this, where the light-exposed parts, areas subject to friction, the flexures and the palmar creases are especially dark. Cushing's disease and ACTH therapy may produce similar changes.

Haemochromatosis is due to a disturbance in iron metabolism leading to the deposition of iron and melanin and producing diffuse bronzing of the skin. Liver disease and diabetes mellitus are also associated. *Biliary cirrhosis*, a disease of middle-aged and elderly women, leads to pigmentation and itching. *Vagabond's disease* presents with pigmentation and also irritation. It is due to body lice and lack of soap and water.

Metallic pigmentation is less frequent than formerly. Inorganic arsenic (Fowler's solution) produces rain drop pigmentation which is a pattern of light coloured macules on a darkened background. Silver, used as eye drops, nose drops, throat sprays and recently anti-smoking lozenges, produces a grey colour more marked in the light-exposed areas. Mercury, which was used extensively in ointments in the past, also produces pigmentation and may still be encountered in industry. Gold pigmentation, chrysiasis, is blue-

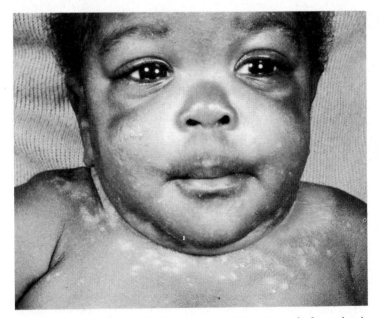

Fig. 93. A baby sent for consultation because of white patches on the face and neck.

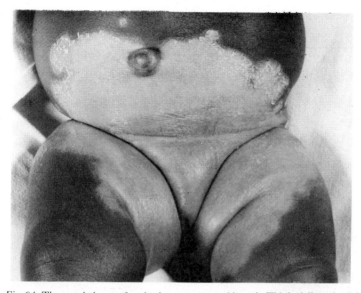

Fig. 94. The same baby was found to have a severe napkin rash. This had disseminated into infantile seborrhoeic dermatitis, hence the appearance in Fig. 93.

grey and is accentuated on light-exposed areas; it is a consequence of gold injections. Drugs may alter the colour of the skin, for example mepacrine gives a yellow colour, β-carotene or an excess of carrots produces carotenaemia, a warm orange colour especially marked on the palms and soles, lamprene (clofazimine) produces a red colour, and chlorpromazine, in a large prolonged dosage, a grey or purple colour.

The latest treatment for psoriasis, 8-methoxypsoralen with longwave ultra-violet light (PUVA), produces an expensive tan. Fixed drug eruptions leave a long-lasting localized pigmentation (see Chapter 11). Inflammation in eczema, lichen planus, impetigo and pityriasis rosea often produces pigmentation in those with dark skin.

Porphyria and pellagra may present with inflammation and pigmentation of the exposed skin. *Chloasma* is pigmentation of the cheeks, forehead and chin. It is a feature of pregnancy and a side effect of the pill. A similar condition, melasma, may develop in Asian and African males.

Genetic and naevoid pigmentation and melanoma

Freckles are small brown-black areas which occur in the summer on the light-exposed parts. They are most evident in children and red-heads. The melanocytes are not more numerous but are larger and more active than normal.

Lentigo (plural lentigenes) is a macule similar to a freckle, but occurring equally on covered parts and commoner in adults. They do not fade in winter. The melanocytes are increased in number.

Café au lait patches are often larger than freckles and lentigenes (Fig. 95). They and axillary 'freckles' are a feature of neurofibromatosis (see Chapter 4), but also occur independently.

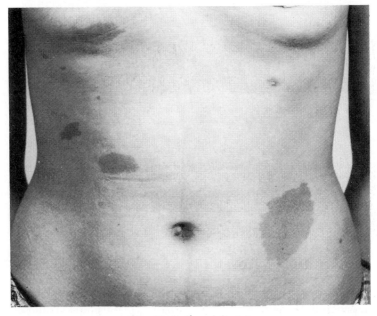

Fig. 95. Café au lait *spots.*

Moles or melanocytic naevi are unusual at birth but become common in childhood and young adult life. They often begin as brown or black macules, called junctional naevi, with an increase in the melanocytes at the dermo-epidermal junction. In many cases the pigment cells drop down into the dermis and produce dermal or compound (dermo-epidermal) naevi. These are the soft moles, called naevus mollis, which are so common on the face and trunk and limbs of adults. They may be skin colour or brown, and frequently have hairs growing from them. These lesions are essentially benign and are usually treated for cosmetic reasons only. Sudden showers of pigmented naevi occur in young people and sometimes in pregnancy. The majority of moles can be left without treatment but is it usual to advise that junctional naevi exposed to recurrent trauma should be excised. Some infants are born with extensive darkly pigmented naevi which later become hairy (bear-skin naevus). These should be removed bit by bit and grafted for they carry a risk of malignancy.

Malignant melanoma

Malignant melanoma represents one per cent of all cancers. They are very rare in infancy and children, unusual in young adults and like most cancers affect the middle-aged and elderly predominantly. Perhaps 50% arise from existing moles, usually the junctional type. Hairy moles are very unlikely to become malignant. Most adults have from 10 – 20 pigmented naevi but only one in a million undergoes metaplasia. Prolonged exposure to the sun is a precipitating factor in whites.

One sign of malignant change is the development of colour irregularities with shades of brown, whitish grey, pink, blue and bluish red occurring. Irregularity of contour both horizontal and vertical (Plate X) is often a feature.

Sudden enlargement, sudden darkening, softening and friability, tenderness, itching or pain are also warning signs. Ulceration and the development of satellites are late signs. Not all melanomas are obviously pigmented and the growing papule, nodule or ulcer should always be examined meticulously for a trace of pigmentation and even this may be absent. In case of doubt, an excision biopsy should be performed for small lesions, and a biopsy for larger ones. Pigmented basal cell carcinoma, seborrhoeic warts and angiomas can all be mistaken for melanomas.

Nodular melanomas, which have a tendency to deep penetration, have the worst prognosis. The superficial spreading melanoma and the melanoma arising from lentigo maligna are less malignant. Lentigo maligna presents as a brownish or blackish

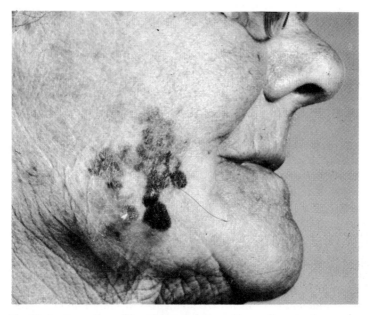

Fig. 96. Lentigo maligna. The nodule at the lower end is a malignant melanoma (see also Plate X).

area of macular pigmentation usually in older people and often on the face (Fig. 96).

Melanomas may occur anywhere on the skin but sun-exposed areas are especially prone. The back is a frequent site in males, the legs in females. Melanomas occur in the perineum, on the soles and palms and underneath the nails. The treatment is excision with a margin from 3–5 cm, depending on the depth of the lesion laterally, and below down to the deep fascia. Skin grafting is almost always needed to fill the defect. The regional lymphnodes should not be removed unless they are involved. Lentigo maligna in the pre-melanomatous stage is treated by excision with a 0.5 cm margin. Immunotherapy and chemotherapy for melanoma are still in the experimental stage.

25

ACNE VULGARIS, ROSACEA, PERI-ORAL DERMATITIS

ACNE VULGARIS

Acne is one of the commonest of the diseases of skin. Because it is mainly a disease of adolescence it has attracted less interest than it deserves until recently, and because it does not threaten life or limb its efficient treatment is often neglected. In fact, the sum of unhappiness directly caused in young people by acne is enormous and its successful treatment gratifies both patient and physician.

Pathogenesis

Acne vulgaris is a chronic disorder of the pilo-sebaceous apparatus, particularly in the skin of the brow, face, shoulders and upper trunk. It is characterized by the formation of excessive amounts of sebum, by obstruction of its outflow and by chemical changes in the retained sebum with the consequent production of inflammatory fatty acids. Rupture of the swollen pilo-sebaceous unit then leads to escape of these materials into the surrounding dermis or sub-cutis, provoking an inflammatory tissue reaction.

True seborrhoea, or excessive production of sebum, has been demonstrated to be a feature of acne subjects when their sebum output is compared with suitably matched controls. The cause of the seborrhoea is debatable. Sebaceous glands are under the control of the sex hormones, the androgenic ones stimulating increased gland size and sebum production, and the oestrogenic ones having an antagonistic effect. Although acne is a feature of syndromes characterized by excessive circulating androgens, e.g. Cushing's and Stein-Leventhal syndromes, the bulk of acne sufferers do not have raised circulating androgen levels. An explanation may be provided by the recent discovery that testosterone can be metabolized in the skin to the more active dihydrotestosterone, a reduction catalysed by the enzyme, 5-α-reductase. This supports the hypothesis that excessive androgenic activity may develop locally around the sebaceous glands and possibly about the hair follicles in 'idiopathic' female hirsutism. Increased levels of dihydrotestosterone have been demonstrated in females with severe acne.

The reasons for the obstruction to outflow are also complex. The amount of sebum, its viscosity, the degree of stratum corneum hydration, and poral hyperkeratosis induced by androgens may all be important. Certainly the comedone, or blackhead, acting like a bath plug, is not a simple cause of obstruction; indeed, its formation may be a consequence rather than a cause of the sluggish sebum flow.

The chemical changes within the retained sebum are better understood because such sebum can be obtained and analysed. Normal sebum consists mainly of triglycerides with smaller amounts of fatty acids, cholesterol, lecithin and phospho-lipids. Retained acne sebum contains a higher than normal proportion of free fatty acids. Almost certainly, these fatty acids are derived from the breakdown of neutral triglycerides by lipases released by the commensal bacterial residents of the pilo-sebaceous unit, namely *Corynebacterium acnes* and *Staphylococcus albus*. However, it has not been convincingly shown that the commensal flora of the acne patient differ quantitatively or qualitatively from the normal.

Trauma by squeezing, damming back of sebum and irritant fatty acids probably all contribute to gland rupture and the consequent fierce, chemically induced inflammation.

Pathology

The lesions of acne are pleomorphic, falling into three groups. Blackheads, or comedones, consist of masses of cornified cells arranged somewhat like the layers of an onion and enclosing inspissated sebum and perhaps a vellus hair. The external part is black due to the presence of melanin. Whiteheads are distended sebaceous glands without a pore. Acne cysts are larger, deeper masses of retained sebum.

All the above are essentially non-inflammatory. The second category of lesions is the consequence of inflammation and includes papules, pustules and abscesses. Post-inflammatory scars of various types constitute the third type of lesion.

Clinical picture

Acne begins at puberty when hormonal activity wakens the latent sebaceous glands of childhood. The peak of incidence is in the years of adolescence but the disease is by no means uncommon in the twenties, nor rare in the thirties. In adolescence the sexes are equally affected, but later the disease is increasingly a problem of women. The face, including the brow, shoulders, nape of neck and the upper trunk in a V-shape are the sites involved although the disease may be localized in any of these areas.

In early adolescence, blackheads and whiteheads often predominate, without obvious inflammation and with only very superficial pin-head papules and pustules. Such acne can nevertheless leave distressing scarring. In more inflammatory disease, the above are combined with larger papules, pustules, abscesses and cysts. Sebo-pus may track to produce elongated fluctuant abscesses (Fig. 97). Occasionally the disease is fulminant, reducing the face and upper trunk of the hapless patient to a florid mass of pleomorphic lesions. Such acne, if allowed to progress, may leave grossly disfiguring and irreversible scarring. Fortunately, some scarring is reversible and the younger the patient the better the prognosis in this regard. If the disease persists after adolescence, blackheads tend to be less evident and the disease tends to become more monomorphic.

The clinical evidence of the seborrhoea is very variable. Patients may complain that the affected skin in whole or in part is very greasy and direct questioning usually, but not always, elicits the fact that the hair has to be washed every two or three days because of its oiliness.

Treatment

The prognosis is a function of the natural severity and longevity of the disease process and the efficacy of treatment. Management depends entirely on the severity of the disease but a long-term view must always be taken. Diet is probably irrelevant but many acne patients insist otherwise and selective withdrawal of sweets, chocolates and cream from the diet is beneficial for other reasons and need not be discouraged by the physician. The affected parts should be washed with ordinary soap not more than twice daily and squeezing of lesions should be strongly discouraged. Ultra-

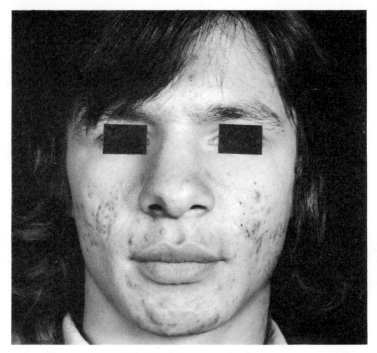

Fig. 97. Severe acne vulgaris.

violet light is usually helpful whether natural, when the climate allows, or artificial.

Topical applications of some use include preparations containing sulphur, benzoyl peroxide (Benoxyl Lotion℞, U.K., U.S.A.), retinoic acid (Retin A lotion℞ or gel, U.K., U.S.A.) and erythromycin. A large number of proprietary lotions, creams, gels and pastes weave variations and combinations on these themes.

If topical therapy has failed, systemic therapy on a long term basis is needed where more than mild inflammation is present. Tetracyclines in a dosage of 250 mg twice a day is the treatment of choice. The effect often builds up slowly so that an eight week initial trial is mandatory. Long term treatment in a dosage of 250 mg twice daily or daily can be continued as long as is necessary. The drug should be taken on an empty stomach and at least half an hour before a meal. Milk and milk products interfere with the absorption of tetracycline as does oral iron. Pregnancy, or possible pregnancy, is an absolute contra-indication to tetracycline therapy and girls must be warned accordingly.

If a two months trial of tetracycline has failed, erythromycin 250 mg twice a day or co-trimoxazole (Septrin, U.K.; Bactrim[R], U.K., U.S.A.) one tablet twice a day can be tried in turn. Either can safely be continued on a long term basis. Probably all of these antibiotic substances act by inhibiting the lipase-producing commensal bacteria of the pilo-sebaceous follicles. They are suppressive and not curative and, if disease activity remains, relapse will follow withdrawal of the drug.

One of these three drugs will control acne in 90% of patients if supported by suitable topical therapy. Occasionally, severe and persistent acne in females, resistant to all other treatment, requires the administration of a high oestrogen oral contraceptive preparations such as Conovid E (U.K.) or Enovid E[R] (U.S.A.), but the physician should be certain there is no gynaecological or other contra-indication to this treatment. Locally applied oestrogen cream is useless.

ACNEIFORM ERUPTIONS

There are a number of clinical situations in which eruptions resembling acne vulgaris may be seen. Drug-induced acne is mentioned in Chapter 11. Steroid-induced acne tends to involve the neck and shoulders more than the face and to be a monomorphic papulo-pustular eruption without comedones. Acne due to isoniazid may be more florid and does involve the face. The muzzle eruption of tuberose sclerosis, misnamed adenoma sebaceum, is acneiform and is seen at puberty (see p. 42).

ROSACEA

Rosacea is a disease of unknown aetiology characterized by an eruption of the central areas of the brow, face and chin and consisting of acneiform papulo-pustules on a background of erythema and telangiectasia. It is seen in both sexes in middle and late life and may be complicated by connective tissue and sebaceous hyperplasia of the nose, particularly in elderly men, and by kerato-conjunctivitis.

Pathogenesis

Both cutaneous blood vessels and the sebaceous glands seem to be involved in rosacea. An abnormal tendency to vasodilatation could explain the observed association with migraine. The response of the papulo-pustular element to small doses of tetracycline suggests that mechanisms similar to those in acne vulgaris may be relevant, a view reinforced by the occasional overlap of acne vulgaris and rosacea in young adults. No pathogenic organism has been demonstrated nor any association with a systemic abnormality, gastro-intestinal or otherwise.

Clinical picture

Rosacea is seen in both sexes. It rarely appears before the fourth decade and the peak of incidence is in the fifth decade. With rare exceptions, the disease is strictly confined to the face, particularly the middle longitudinal third, i.e. the central forehead, nose and cheeks and chin. A tendency to flush easily may be an early symptom. Later the affected areas become increasingly red and large telangiectatic venules are seen, especially on the nose and cheeks. Papules of varying sizes or papulo-pustules develop in some patients (Plate XII). Rhinophyma is an uncommon complication, seen almost exclusively in elderly men in which sebaceous and connective tissue proliferation occurs in the nose, occasionally producing a grotesque deformity (Fig. 98).

Rosacea is a chronic disorder which may persist for years or even decades although varying in severity.

An iatrogenic variant of the disease has become increasingly common in the last decade due to the use of potent fluorinated corticosteroids in treatment. The picture of a smooth atrophic skin, severe telangiectasia and crops of papulo-pustules occurring especially when the treatment is temporarily stopped is characteristic (see also Peri-oral Dermatitis below).

Management

Tetracycline by mouth in very small dosage is the treatment of choice. Almost always 250 mg twice daily promptly suppresses the papulo-pustular component of the disease and control can be maintained by 250 mg once daily or even once every second day. The telangiectatic element is less easy to treat but often improves with long term tetracycline treatment.

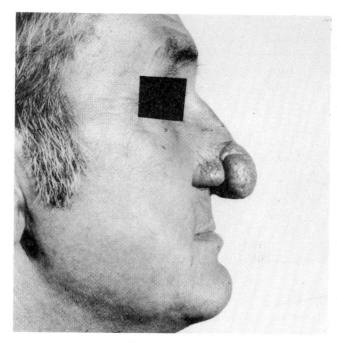

Fig. 98. Rhinophyma.

Topical preparations are of limited value. Hydrocortisone acetate as a 1% cream or 0.5% sulphur in an aqueous cream may
sometimes be useful. Potent corticosteroids should never be used.
If the patient presents on such steroids, they must be withdrawn,
tetracycline started orally and the patient warned that the disease
will get worse for up to 10 days before improving. Diet, hormonal
therapy and other systemic measures are of no value.

The disease is chronic for decades in some patients but is phasic
in others, settling spontaneously.

PERI-ORAL DERMATITIS

This label has been applied to a clinical picture which has come to
prominence in the last 15 years and is thought to be mainly but not
entirely iatrogenic.

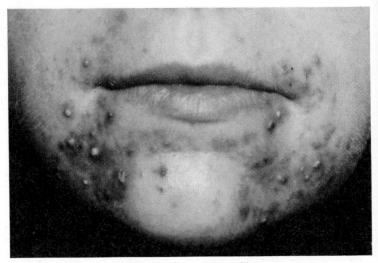

Fig. 99. Peri-oral dermatitis.

Clinical picture

The patient is almost always female, in the third, fourth or fifth decades of life, and presents with a striking peri-oral eruption of small papulo-pustules. Usually there is also erythema, telangiectasia and atrophy of the skin with the same distribution as that of a potent fluorinated steroid cream that has been applied daily for months or even years (Fig. 99). Comedones are absent. Such a therapeutic history is almost always obtained, the treatment usually having been started for trivial reasons and continued indefinitely because of the subjective satisfaction obtained. Direct questioning also generally elicits the story that temporary withdrawal of the steroid cream results in rapid 'deterioration' of the skin of the face, leading to prompt restoration of treatment.

Rarely, the peri-oral eruption is seen in the absence of such a history and it is a matter of debate whether it then constitutes a localized variant of rosacea.

Management

Treatment is identical with that for steroid aggravated rosacea. After temporary worsening the prognosis is excellent and the peri-oral skin has usually returned to normal within three months.

26

DISEASES OF THE NAILS

The structure of nail, the nail fold and nail bed is described on page 14. Abnormalities of these structures may be congenital or acquired. The former are all rare.

CONGENITAL NAIL DYSTROPHIES

Nail patella syndrome

This syndrome is inherited as a mendelian dominant triat. The nails are absent or rudimentary. Not all digits are necessarily involved but thumb changes are always found. The patella is palpably small or absent.

Pachyonychia congenita

In this disorder the nails become thickened and hyperkeratotic and there may be associated keratoderma and other muco-cutaneous changes.

Dystrophic epidermolysis bullosa

Nail dystrophy is characteristic of this inherited disease in which the skin blisters readily in response to trauma.

Other defects occasionally seen are complete absence of nails (anonychia) or severe dystrophies as part of widespread ectodermal dysplasias. Leuconychia (white nails), onycholysis (separation of nail plate from its bed), koilonychia (spoon-shaped nails) and clubbing are all occasionally seen soon after birth.

ACQUIRED NAIL DYSTROPHIES

Infections

Tinea unguium and candidiasis are described in Chapter 7.

Onycholysis of any cause may be complicated by Gram-negative proliferation in the nail bed, often due to *Pseudomonas aeruginosa* which may cause a greenish discoloration of the lifted nail plate. Paronychia (infection of the nail fold) may be acute or chronic. The acute condition is pyococcal, developing rapidly after infection of a nail fold cut or abrasion into a painful, tender, fluctuant paronychial abscess. Surgical drainage alone may be curative but an appropriate antibiotic may be added to hasten cure.

Chronic paronychia

Chronic paronychia is a common and important condition in which candidial infection is one factor. It is usually seen in women whose hands are constantly in water, e.g. barmaids, kitchen and canteen workers, and housewives with young children, but men in occupations carrying the same hazard, e.g. chefs, are equally at risk. Ischaemia as in progressive systemic sclerosis predisposes to chronic paronychia.

The initial change is maceration and then separation of the nail fold (cuticle) from the nail plate. Irritants such as soap, detergents and food, and micro-organisms then enter the sub-cuticular space leading to inflammation, manifesting as a red tender swelling (bolstering) of the nail fold. Cheesy material may be discharged from this space. As the inflammation persists the emerging nail becomes abnormal, ridged horizontally, roughened and often discoloured (see Fig. 37). Treatment consists of encouraging the patient to keep the hands dry by use of gloves for wet work. Local applications with anti-candidal or anti-bacterial activity may be helpful such as 1% aqueous gentian violet, 1:5000 potassium permanganate, nystatin ointment, amphotericin B lotion or Tri-Adcortyl cream (U.K.). Griseofulvin is of no value.

Nail dystrophy due to trauma

Nail biting takes many forms leading to different deformities. Biting or rubbing of the posterior nail fold may lead to severe ridging of the nail. Subungual haematoma is important since it occasionally leads to suspicion of malignant melanoma of the nail bed. Tight shoes may be a factor causing ingrowing toe nails.

Chemical trauma is a much less common cause of nail dystrophy. It may be seen in engineering workers due to oils. Damage due to nail varnishes and related chemicals is rare. Drug reactions involving the nails are also rare. Tetracyclines can cause a photo-onycholysis and the colour of the nail may be changed to yellow by tetracycline, grey-blue by argyria and blue-black by chloroquine.

Skin diseases

Many skin diseases affect the nails. Psoriatic nail changes are described on page 193. If eczema affects the distal finger, secondary ridging of the nail is common. Lichen planus (p. 201) and alopecia areata (p. 254) can all affect the nail in characteristic fashion.

Miscellaneous dystrophies

Identical horizontal ridged defects across all the nails indicate a transient interuption of nail growth (Beau's lines). Severe illness of many types can also be responsible.

Koilonychia, or spoon-shaped nails, is classically seen in iron deficiency but also occurs in lichen planus and may be congenital.

Finger clubbing involves the increased curvature of the nail in both directions and loss of the angle between the cuticle and nail. The common causes are chronic lung disease or cyanotic heart disease but it may be seen in thyroid disease, biliary cirrhosis and ulcerative colitis.

Yellow nail syndrome is due to a disorder of lymphatic drainage in the limb. The nails are thick, yellow, curved and grow very slowly.

Splinter haemorrhages are seen in many dermatological and general medical conditions such as trauma, psoriasis, rheumatoid arthritis, infective endocarditis and collagen diseases.

Onycholysis is the separation of the nail plate from its bed. It is often idiopathic and involves all or most of the finger nails, sometimes for many years.

Coloured half-moons. The half-moon (lunula) may be red in heart failure and brown in chronic renal failure.

27

DISORDERS OF THE SCALP AND HAIR

ALOPECIA

Alopecia means loss of hair. It is convenient to divide the causes of alopecia as in Fig. 100.

THE SCARRING (CICATRICIAL) ALOPECIAS

These are conditions in which damage to the scalp skin by trauma or inflammation destroys hair follicles causing irreversible hair loss (Fig. 101). The traumatic causes include thermal, chemical and radiation burns. The inflammatory diseases which do so are discoid lupus erythematosus, lichen planus, zoster affecting the first division of the trigeminal nerve and, very rarely these days, lupus vulgaris and tertiary syphilis. The rare chronic fungal infection called favus also does so (see p. 81).

LOCALIZED NON-SCARRING ALOPECIA

This pattern of hair loss is generally due to alopecia areata, tinea capitis or trauma. Secondary syphilis is a rare cause of patchy 'moth-eaten' alopecia. Tinea capitis is described on p. 80. Relevant trauma may be pulling or twisting out of hair by nervous children or psychotic adults. Traction may be from combs or plaits and is common in black women after straightening procedures when it tends to cause a marginal alopecia (Fig. 102). Persistent nervous rubbing may fracture hairs to produce areas of stubbly hair loss.

Alopecia areata

This is an extremely common condition characterized by complete hair loss from patches of the scalp. It has a rapid onset but a strong tendency to spontaneous reversal.

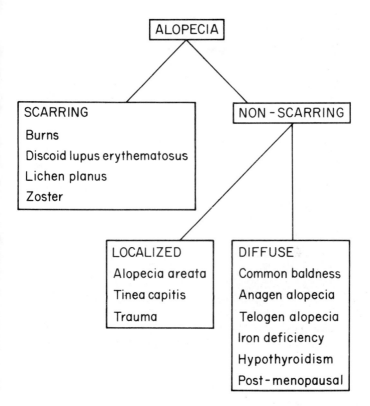

Fig. 100. A simplified classification of alopecia.

The condition is of unknown aetiology but there appears to be an ill-defined genetic factor. There is a clinical association with vitiligo, in which organ-specific autoantibodies may be found, but there is no direct evidence that alopecia areata itself is due to autoimmune mechanisms. Some atopic subjects develop alopecia areata and in such cases the prognosis for regrowth is poor.

The disease may first appear at any age but usually does so in the second or third decades, affecting both sexes equally. Sharply defined bald patches of any size develop rapidly. Usually there are no local symptoms but itching and slight tenderness may be elicited. The disease is rarely total on the scalp or universal, affecting

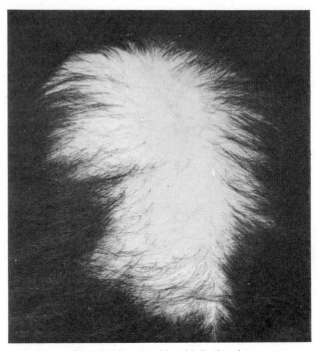

Fig. 101. Scarring (cicatricial) alopecia.

every hair follicle on the body including eyebrows and eyelashes
(Fig. 103).

On examination the affected skin looks normal. Sometimes
dystrophic 'exclamation-mark' hairs are seen especially at the
margins of lesions (Fig. 104). These are very short broken hairs,
tapering and becoming depigmented as the scalp is approached.
Plucking reveals such hairs to be in the telogen phase (see p. 11).
Pitting of the finger nails may also be seen.

In the localized forms of the disease, the prognosis is generally
for complete recovery to occur after many weeks or even months.
When the hair does regrow it is usually depigmented at first but
later hair growth is completely normal. The prognosis is poor
when alopecia areata is extensive around the ears and posterior
scalp (opheasic pattern). It is also poor when total or universal

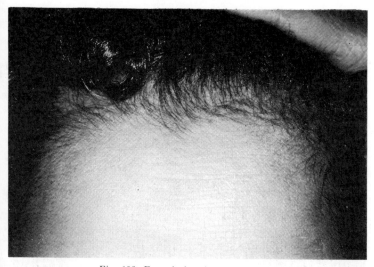

Fig. 102. Frontal alopecia due to traction.

alopecia develops in early life. Nevertheless, potential follicular function is retained even after decades of inactivity as can be demonstrated by local steroid injection. Such local steroid therapy, given by needle injection or 'spray gun', is the only effective form of treatment but its results are only temporary and it is only appropriate or possible in localized disease. Topical application of steroids, oestrogens, etc. have no effect. In severe forms of the disease the patient may wish to resort to a wig.

DIFFUSE NON-SCARRING ALOPECIAS

Common baldness

The signs of this condition, also known as male pattern alopecia, need no description. The rate and extent of balding are controlled by genetic factors and the patient's age. Adequate levels of circulating androgens are a pre-requisite for these factors to operate and this is probably the main factor protecting pre-menopausal females since the administration of androgens to women may lead to balding at the temples and crown, giving the so-called android pattern of hair loss. No treatment can reverse the condition. Only

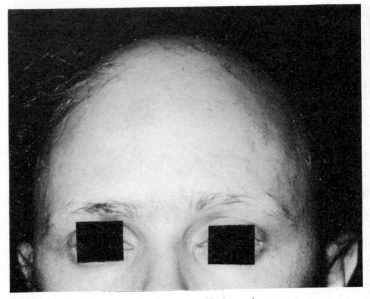

Fig. 103. Alopecia areata affecting eyebrows.

castration will arrest its progress. Transplantation of hair-bearing grafts from non-balding areas of the scalp is the only effective treatment but this is only an impressive cosmetic procedure in highly skilled and expensive hands.

Anagen alopecia

This is the result of therapy with antimitotic drugs for malignant disease. The anagen follicle is vulnerable to such agents and produces a dystrophic hair which breaks soon after emerging from the scalp. Cyclophosphamide and methotrexate are well-recognized causes.

Telogen alopecia

Certain stresses can prematurely switch anagen follicles into the telogen phase without doing further damage. The event is masked until about three months later when large numbers of these follicles synchronously switch back into a new anagen phase, resulting in the loss of the resting, telogen, hair. This produces a hair fall

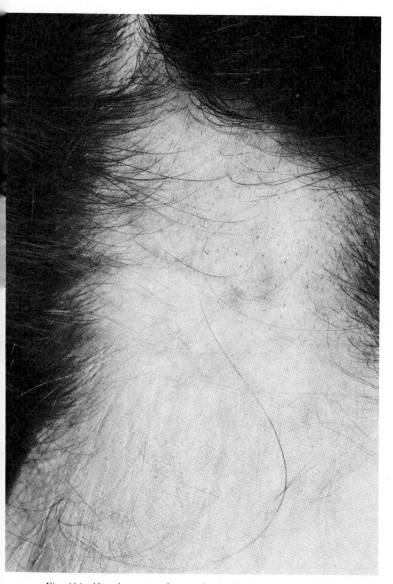

Fig. 104. Alopecia areata of nape, showing 'exclamation mark' hairs.

whose severity is precisely proportional to the number of affected follicles.

The stress factors which may be responsible include childbirth (post-partum alopecia), severe acute infection (post-infective alopecia), withdrawal of oral contraceptive tablets (usually mild) and 'crash' dieting. Severe psychological stress may also act similarly as may anti-coagulant and anti-thyroid drugs.

Prognosis is excellent but, in severe cases, temporary use of a wig may be necessary.

Metabolic alopecia

Severe iron deficiency at any age can cause diffuse hair loss (Fig. 105) as may hypothyroidism. The cause is confirmed by the appropriate laboratory tests. Less frequently hyperthyroidism and the connective tissue diseases may be incriminated.

Post-menopausal alopecia

This is probably the female equivalent of male balding modified by the differing endocrine conditions and possibly different genetic mechanisms. As in the male, it is enormously variable.

Idiopathic pre-menopausal alopecia

This is a common condition and may begin as early as the third decade. There is never, by definition, any overt endocrinopathy but sophisticated studies of sex-hormone metabolism may reveal abnormalities in a minority. Hypothyroidism and iron deficiency must be excluded with certainty because the disease causes great unhappiness and there is no safe effective treatment. High-oestrogen oral contraceptives may sometimes arrest the process but their use carries a low but definite risk of thrombo-embolism particularly in women over 35 years and in heavy smokers.

HIRSUTIES (HYPERTRICHOSIS)

The name hirsuties, or hypertrichosis, signifies an excessive or abnormal development of hair on areas of the body which normally only bear vellus hairs. The condition may be congenital or acquired, localized or diffuse. Occasionally the word hypertrichosis is used when referring to abnormally luxuriant growths of hair occurring on areas such as the eyebrows or eyelids which normally bear hair.

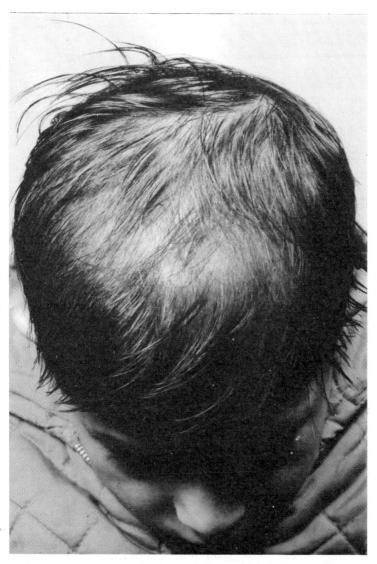

Fig. 105. *Diffuse non-scarring alopecia in a child, associated with severe nutritional iron deficiency anaemia.*

Congenital hirsuties

The infant may be covered with hair, or the abnormal growth may be confined to a relatively small area. In many of the cases the hair develops on a large deeply pigmented mole, and the abnormality then persists throughout the whole of the patient's life. Abnormal tufts of hair which are not associated with mole formation frequently fall out shortly after birth and are replaced by normal vellus hairs. Children suffering from this complaint usually exhibit other congenital deformities, e.g. cleft palate or spina bifida. A long tail of hair arising from the lumbar lesion is the commonest presenting symptom of spina bifida.

Acquired hirsuties

Acquired hirsuties is more common in females than in males, and usually occurs in localized areas, especially on the chin and upper lip; the condition frequently develops at puberty and after the climacteric. The majority of cases are believed to be due to endocrine dysfunction, but if hirsuties commences during adolescence, and if there are no other stigmata of endocrine dysfunction, the condition will not usually be influenced by endocrine therapy. If there is adiposity, hypertension or other features, steps must be taken to exclude an adrenal or ovarian tumour. Basophil adenoma of the pituitary (Cushing's syndrome) is associated with hairiness of the face and trunk in women, but with hairlessness in males. In the Stein-Leventhal syndrome there are lutein cysts in both ovaries and their capsules are thickened; this is associated with infertility, amenorrhoea or oligomenorrhoea, and sometimes with obesity and hirsutism. Porphyria cutanea tarda causes hypertrichosis in both sexes.

Treatment

If the hypertrichosis occurs on an area which is covered by clothes, the condition is best left untreated. Small, pigmented, hairy areas may be excised. Dark hair may be bleached and made less conspicuous by applying a freshly prepared stiff paste made of Fuller's earth or kaolin and 30 volume hydrogen peroxide and a few drops of ammonia. The paste should be washed off after 5 or 10 minutes. In severe cases depilating creams, epilatory wax, razors or pumice-stone may be used. In skilled hands treatment with electrolysis gives good results, but care must be taken lest unsightly scars are produced. In most cases a good, cosmetic, depilating cream is the treatment of choice.

INGROWING HAIRS OF THE BEARD

This is a common disease of black men due to tight curling of the beard hair but may occur in Caucasians especially if a very close shave is obtained with the skin tightly stretched. The free end of the hair, sharpened by shaving, penetrates the skin either inside or beyond the follicle. As it pushes into the skin a foreign body inflammatory response occurs producing a characteristic papular reaction. In blacks, papular keloids may follow forming acne keloid (Fig. 106).

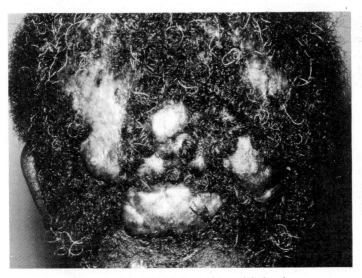

Fig. 106. Acne keloid lesions of the occipital scalp.

Differential diagnosis is from staphylococcal folliculitis. Treatment is not easy nor very effective. Close shaving should be avoided and growing a beard may help. Ingrowing hairs should be pulled out.

28

DISORDERS OF THE SWEAT GLANDS

Excessive production of sweat can be localized or diffuse, transient or chronic. Its distribution depends upon the cause. Many systemic disorders may cause hyperhidrosis. These include neurological lesions, particularly in the pontine, medullary and cervical areas; endocrinopathies such as hyperthyroidism; infections causing periodic abnormal temperature variations and metabolic upsets such as insulin-induced hypoglycaemia or, rarely, phaeochromocytoma. Gustatory hyperhidrosis i.e. sweating on the lips, forehead and nose, may be induced by eating hot spicy foods and is usually physiological; rarely, pathological gustatory sweating may be due to disease of the autonomic nervous system or disturbances of the parotid gland.

Notwithstanding this long list of causes, hyperhidrosis is usually idiopathic. It is most commonly encountered in the second and third decade and in either sex. The hands especially the palms and axillae are the commonest sites of troublesome sweating but patients may complain of hyperhidrosis of the feet or face. Anogenital hyperhidrosis seems to be common in middle-aged men whose lives are stressful e.g. business executives. There is no doubt that mental or emotional stress evokes sweating of palms, soles and axillae, which can be simply demonstrated. Such stress can also evoke sweating of the forehead, nose, mid-lines of the chest and the back in some individuals; indeed generalized sweating may occasionally be provoked in this way. However, in many young people minimal physical or mental activity is sufficient to produce palmar or axillary sweating, e.g. ordinary social intercourse. In a few unfortunate young people such sweating is almost continuous and may be related to obvious or occult emotional disorders.

Fortunately the long term prognosis for emotional or idiopathic hyperhidrosis is good, and the condition eventually disappears. Typically onset is soon after puberty and the condition has cleared by the age of 20–25 years.

Treatment. Management is unsatisfactory. Commercial anti-perspirants containing aluminium salts may be useful in mild cases. Aqueous formaldehyde may be useful on the soles, applied as soaks daily for 15 minutes. The best treatment for the axillae is 20% aluminium chloride hexahydrate in 70% alcohol, painted on at night and washed off in the morning.

Glycopyrronium bromide (Robinul, U.K.) is the most useful oral anti-perspirant. Its anti-cholinergic action may result in side effects, particularly a dry mouth. In a dosage of 2 – 4 mg once or twice daily it can suppress sweating for up to six hours successfully. Propantheline bromide (Probanthine, U.K.) 15 – 30 mg is less useful.

In severe intractable axillary hyperhidrosis, resistant to medical measures, surgical excision of the sweat-gland bearing skin is effective but leaves a cosmetically unpleasant scar and sometimes some limitation of shoulder movement. It should only rarely be necessary. Cervical sympathectomy abolishes palmar sweating but surgery is best avoided in what is usually a self-limiting disease.

ANHIDROSIS

This is the absence of sweating even after local pharmacological provocation. It is often unnoticed by the patient but may lead to heat intolerance or itching. Anhidrosis may be congenital as part of an ectodermal dysplasia. Acquired causes include peripheral neuritis e.g. in leprosy or diabetes, a variety of systemic diseases such as myxoedema, Addison's disease and Sjogren's syndrome, and certain skin diseases, particularly psoriasis and erythroderma. It may be chemically induced, topically by formaldehyde or glutaraldehyde or systemically as in mepacrine-induced lichenoid eruptions.

BROMHIDROSIS

This is an abnormal or excessive skin odour. Apocrine bromhidrosis is an axillary problem and is due to decomposition of apocrine sweat by surface bacteria; management consists of frequent washing and the local use of antibacterial agents, e.g. chlorhexidine (Hibitane Cream, U.K.). Eccrine bromhidrosis, induced by the activity of bacteria on sweat-sodden stratum corneum in the feet, can lead to a highly offensive odour. Soap and water are reasonably effective especially in male patients who have previously practised excessive restraint in their use.

MILIARIA (PRICKLY HEAT)

This is an acute eruption characterized by itching and the development of a papular, vesicular or pustular eruption. It is caused by sweat duct blockage induced by tropical heat and humidity or similar conditions engendered by excessive activity in unsuitable clothing, e.g. by troops in less extreme climates. Probably over-hydration of the stratum corneum is the immediate cause of the sweat duct occlusion.

Treatment includes the encouragement of sweat evaporation by the provision, where possible, of appropriate environmental conditions such as air conditioning and clothing. Ascorbic acid 1 g orally daily may be of prophylactic value.

HIDRADENITIS SUPPURATIVA

This is a rare condition in which recurrent and later chronic infection involves the apocrine apparatus, usually in one or both axillae but sometimes in the ano-genital folds. The clinical signs vary from recurrent transient follicular papules to boils, abscesses, sinus formation, scarring and fibrosis. Antibiotics are of limited value and extensive surgery or radiotherapy may be needed for advanced cases. The disease may last for decades.

APPENDIX

LOCAL CORTICOSTEROID PREPARATIONS

Corticosteroids currently available are legion. We have listed only a few. These have been divided into the following categories: very strong, strong, medium, and weak. In principle one chooses the weakest steroid which will produce the desired result. Most of these preparations are available as ointment, cream, lotion or scalp lotion. In general, an ointment produces a stronger effect than the equivalent cream or lotion because of the occlusive effect of its base. Ointments can be diluted with soft paraffin which can save a lot of money. Money can also be saved by choosing a cheaper preparation which may be just as effective as an expensive one. A cream is often cosmetically more acceptable than an ointment. For the scalp, lotion is the most acceptable. The ordinary lotions do not sting or cause as much drying as the scalp lotions or applications which have an alcoholic vehicle.

Very strong	Beclomethasone dipropionate 0.5% (Propaderm Forte, U.K.)
	Clobestasol propionate 0.05% (Dermovate, U.K.)
	Diflucortolone valerate 0.3% (Nerisone Forte, U.K.)
	Fluocinolone acetonide 0.2% (Synalar Forte, U.K.; Synalar – HP[R], U.S.A.)
Strong	Betamethasone valerate 0.1% (Betnovate, U.K.; Valisone[R], U.S.A.)
	Clobetasol propionate 0.05% (Dermovate, U.K.) diluted 1 in 3 with soft paraffin (ointment only)

Fluocinolone acetonide 0.025%
(Synalar, U.K.; Fluonid^R, U.S.A.)
Triamcinolone acetonide 0.1%
(Adcortyl, U.K.; Aristocort^R or, Kenalog^R,
U.S.A.)

Medium

Betamethasone valerate 0.1%
(Betnovate, U.K.; Valisone^R, U.S.A.)
diluted 1 in 5 with soft paraffin (ointment
only).
Fluocinolone 0.01%
(Synandone, U.K. and weaker strength
Synalar and Fluonid^R, U.S.A.)
Flurandrenolone 0.0125%
(Haelan, U.K.)
Hydrocortisone-17-butyrate 0.1%
(Locoid, U.K.)

Weak

Hydrocortisone 0.5%, 1% and 2.5%

INDEX

F following a page number indicates a figure and T indicates a table